The NHS General Practice

REVOLUTION

Dr. Hamid Sarwar

This edition is published by
Grosvenor Books London 2022

CONTENTS

Acknowledgements

I would like to thank the following eminent people for their help:

Mr. Nigel Edwards
Chief Executive Officer, Nuffield Trust, London.
Mr. Edwards was formerly an expert adviser with KPMG's Global Centre of Excellence for Health and Life Sciences and a Senior Fellow at The King's Fund. He was Policy Director of the NHS Confederation for 11 years. Nuffield Trust is an independent health think tank with the mission of improving health care in the UK through evidence and analyses

Mr. Jamie Kaffash
Editor, Pulse
Awarded Best New Editor
The Fiona MacPherson New Editor award 2019
British Society of Magazine Editors.
Awarded Editor of the year 2020. Medical Journalist Association
Pulse is the publication for the General Practitioners

Dr. Euan Lawson
Editor, British Journal of General Practice
Co-author of books: The Healthy Writer. GP Wellbeing.

Ms. Emma Bower
Editor, GP online. GP Business

Ms Eleni Kyriacou
An award-winning editor and journalist. She has written for The Guardian, Marie Claire, Grazia, You, among others.
Autor of the novel
"She came to stay"

Author's Note

This book deals with the General Practice in England only and not the UK.

I hereby declare that the facts and statistics in this book are correct to the best of my knowledge and ability at the time of writing. To assure an instant verification, I have provided sources of all the statistical information. Here are two examples to explain:

My job is to make sure you don't have to wait three weeks to see your GP (Boris Johnson, Prime minister, July 2019)

Increasing numbers of patients are waiting over three weeks to get a GP appointment, with 11 million having done so since the prime minister pledged to end the delays (Doctors' publication, pulsetoday.co.uk)

I have provided a legally binding written agreement to all the people who have contributed to this book to promise that their names and details will never be divulged to a third party. I have checked the accuracy of the contributor's opinions, without altering their text and avoided those whose comments appeared to be biased or could not be verified. All royalties of this book will be donated to a charity, 'Save Nation's Health'.

After fifteen months of research, comprising three hundred A4 pages, condensed and edited to what you have in this book, I am saddened to say that I have been unable to find aspects of the General Practice in England, which could be seen as genuinely helpful to people seeking medical attention.

The small size of the book is deliberate. It would be stupid if I should claim greatness by the simple act of writing this short book. However great books of this size have been written. My favourite books of around 130 pages

Non-Fiction
The Art of War (Sun Tzu)
The Prince (Niccolò Machiavelli)
The Fire Next Time ((James Baldwin)
The Richest Man in Babylon (George S. Clason)
The Prophet (Kahlil Gibran)
The Lessons of History (Will Durant, Ariel Durant)
The one minute manager (Ken Blanchard)
On the Duty of Civil Disobedience (David Thoreau)

Fiction
Metamorphosis (Franz Kafka)
The Death of Ivan Ilych (Leo Tolstoy)
Death in Venice (Thomas Mann)
Animal Farm (George Orwell)
Candide (Voltaire)
Waiting for Godot (Samuel Beckett)
The Old Man and the Sea (Earnest Hemingway)
Notes from the Underground (Fyodor Dostoyevsky)

I dedicate this book to, the long-suffering people in England.

We suffer because we wait two weeks to get a GP appointment.

We suffer when for 110 hours every week, we are forced to receive treatment by telephone only, from the wholly inadequate NHS 111 Call Centre.

We suffer when driven to the A&E because the GPs do not provide consultations after 6 pm and at the weekends, unlike their hospital colleagues.

My book demonstrates without a reasonable doubt that, 'no wait' 24/7/365 face-to-face GP consultations are achievable both operationally and financially.

This book would act as the 'campaign manual'

The NHS General Practice REVOLUTION

can happen if, all of us campaign to convince the MPs and the Prime minister to accept the book's findings and implement the recommendations through legislation. How can anyone argue with it when no extra funding is required except a modest and affordable sum?

Please note: The website www.nhsrevolution.org is live and interactive to inform you and update the developments related to the 'NHS Revolution Campaign'.

Introduction

The Primary care provided to the people of England through the NHS General Practice is one of the worst in the world when it comes to getting prompt GP appointments. Even then they are denied after 6pm and the weekends. It is so fundamentally flawed that only a "Revolution" can reverse its collapse.'

You have every reason to be startled by the word 'revolution'. A revolution in England? In the NHS General Practice?

I am not referring here to the bloody American, French, Russian, Chinese, Cuban or Iranian revolutions or the Industrial revolution. Let us take a philosophical, intellectual and historical perspective.

It was only during the Renaissance that the revolution as a cause of change was recognised by people like Niccolò Machiavelli (the 16th century Italian writer). His detailed analysis of power, led to a new belief in the necessity of changes in the structure of Government, 'on certain occasions'. John Milton, (the 17th century English writer), believed in the revolution's inherent ability to help realise its full potential. Immanuel Kant, (the 18th century German Philosopher), believed in revolution as a force for the advancement of humankind. The thought process was carried on by Hegel, Marx and later by the scholars like Crane Brinton, Farideh Farhi, Mason Hart, Jack Gladstone, Barrington Moore, Jeffery Paige, Vilfredo Pareto, Carlos Vistas, Eric Wolf, to mention a few.

Even the ancient Greek Philosopher Aristotle (384-322 BC), described two types of political revolution: complete change from one constitution to another and modification of an existing system.

The classical definition of a revolution (*Latin: revolutiq, meaning 'a turnaround'*) implies a fundamental change in political power and organisation, which occurs when the population revolts, due to oppression or political incompetence.

Why a revolution? What would this revolution look like? Riots, chaos, street violence? No. It would be through a gentle, peaceful movement, a relentless, unstoppable campaign to convince the MPs, the politicians, and the Government to 'turnaround'. This would only be achievable through a calm, genial, conciliatory, felicitous revolt by the masses of England.

In this book, I have provided a comprehensive treatise on the continuous deterioration and reasons of failure of the NHS General Practice, which continues to inflict irrefutable misery on the people of England.

More importantly, I have presented a credible, evidence-based solution within the NHS General Practice Budget. One may ask, why everyone does not jump with joy at my implementable solution? It appears that those related to the NHS General Practice are in a narcissistic and egotistical state of denial. The overall view seems to be; 'why bother?'

'Why bother', when the NHS General Practice industry feeds billions of pounds to those running it, those employed in it, those making outlandish hand-outs from it?

'Why bother', when the national and international investors are making a killing from it?

'Why bother', when everyone has been made to believe that the free General Practice 'is the envy of the world'?

'Why bother', when people in England are suffering and dying, without complaining, because they have been brainwashed to believe that it is the duty of the people to 'protect the NHS' and not the duty of the 'NHS to protect the people'?

'Why bother', when the Government finds it easier to sing the praises of the NHS General Practice than identify and rectify the horrendous problems facing the people?

Why bother indeed? Read this book to find out why. What we need now is a total *turnaround*, an actual revolution!

A revolution, of the people, by the people, for the people. A revolution, to throw out the conviction of those running the NHS General Practice that people in England cannot and should not receive face-to-face consultations with the GPs after 6 pm and over the weekends. A revolution to secure an acceptable primary healthcare system.

The WHO constitution envisages:

'Understanding health as a human right creates a legal obligation on states to ensure access to timely, acceptable and affordable health care of appropriate quality'.

The book will show that the Government does not appear to be meeting its human rights obligations to the people of England in providing timely and acceptable healthcare through the NHS General Practice.

Join the 'Revolution' to persuade and convince the MPs of all the political parties and the Government that through the legislation, the General Practice in England should have a 'turnaround, a revolutiq', a Radical Reform to relieve the misery and sufferings of millions of people in England.

Chapter One

A tale of two General Practices: from an age of wisdom to an era of foolishness, from the season of light to the season of darkness, from the spring of hope to the winter of despair. Rise and Fall of the Great English General Practice. Birth of the GP Contractor.

The story of the transformation of General Practice from a genuine world-beating service to the dreadful offering we have today is an example of the incompetence, lack of planning and failure of those at the helm of affairs - the NHS Management.

Let us commence the story, from 1948, when the British General Practice was established along with the NHS. The golden period of the General Practice began in 1948. The beginning of its end started 2004, onwards. The GPs were declared self-employed, though fully paid by the NHS with a legal commitment to offer their services 24/7, throughout the year.

Very quickly, our General Practice became the best in the world. You had your own family doctor, who looked after you and the family, from cradle to grave. Your GP provided instant appointments, delivered babies, provided terminal care and would visit if the person was too ill to attend. All of this was free and available 24/7. The GP was a pillar of the society, much loved and revered.

Every person in the UK was registered in the name of one GP, as a single hand or multiple doctors' practice. The vast majority of all consultations took place with the patient's 'own' doctor except when the latter was on holiday.

To provide a 24/7 service to the people, GPs formed a network rota to provide cover at nights and Saturday 1pm to

Monday 8am, for each other's patients. Most doctors had a Saturday morning surgery session. The mainstay of this model was the contractual commitment by an individual GP to provide treatment and advice to the patients 24/7, if so required.

Because of their availability during this period, any medical problems arising after hours were genuine and dealt with by the GP or a colleague covering nights or weekends.

Apart from major traumas and genuine emergencies, where an ambulance could be called to take a patient to A&E, every medical problem had to be seen by the GP first. If an urgent second opinion or a hospital admission was required, the GP would talk on phone to a relevant doctor on night duty explaining why the patient was being sent to A&E. A handwritten note had to be taken to A&E. The usual practice was for a relative to take the patient in a car or a taxi. An ambulance to transport an otherwise ambulant patient was unheard of.

The duty of care and treatment by the GP for a patient on the practice list was paramount. Anyone receiving attention at night or the weekend was to report to their 'own' GP for a follow-up. The ultimate responsibility to look after a problem that created a night or weekend consultation was that of the GP. Continuity of care was considered essential.

The GPs after forming a network to cover each other at nights and weekends and working say one night in 10 or one weekend in six did not feel it hard. After all, every doctor was accustomed to doing it in hospitals before entering the general practice.

This model of Primary Care in Britain was a genuine 'pride of the nation and envy of the world'. Throughout England, organisations exist which provide 24-hour services, seven days a week, 365 days a year. These are sometimes called "round the clock services" and examples include: A&E, airports, airlines, ambulance, electricity suppliers, fire services, filling stations, hospitals, primary care, police and taxis. Gyms, pubs, restaurants, night clubs and some supermarkets open after 6pm and over the weekends.

It would be unthinkable and frankly impossible for any of the above to have an 'out of hours service' restricted from 8am to 6pm, Monday to Friday.

In 2004, a new contract was introduced for the General Practice, euphemistically called "*Alternative Provider of Medical Services*"*(APMS)*. With the stroke of a pen, the 56-year-old model of the General Practice providing 24/7/365 was converted to a bank clerk, office hours, Monday to Friday model by declaring that any illness that occurred after 6pm and on weekends, was no longer the responsibility of the GPs. The laughable concept of *"out of hours GP services"* was born and GPs were given an option to opt out of providing 24/7 services if they so wished; 100% were glad to do so.

Never, in the history of commercial, private, voluntary, or public enterprises has there been an example where the availability of a workforce has been reduced from 168 to 50 hours a week. GPs are now available from 8am to 6pm. Their Surgeries or Health Centres are open, staffed by receptionists, nurses, managers. The patients your GP is seeing today are those who made appointments 2 weeks ago.

The catastrophic consequences of the reforms of 2004 and that of 2012 Health & Social Care Act have changed the British General Practice as follows:

1. The bank clerk's working hours of a GP with 2 weeks wait to make an appointment has turned the historical British General Practice from 'the envy of the world' to the 'laughingstock of the world'.
2. For 118 hours a week, when your own GP is no longer available, the responsibility of all health problems has been transferred to the so called 'out of hours services '. There is no possibility of continuity of care.
3. The massive 'out of hours' responsibility to look after the people's health problems has added a significant strain on the NHS budget, which is already dwindling. It has also created a money-making opportunity for private companies, which claim to provide an instant face-to-face, video or telephone appointment.
4. Continuity of care and responsibility of follow-up treatment of an individual by their 'own GP' has ceased to exist.
5. Unable to get a GP appointment, people are forced to seek help from the NHS 111 and the A&E department.

The General Practice in England, as it is now, has been described by several analysts as "One of the worst in the world to get a GP appointment." The most devastating outcome of these reforms has been the birth of the GP contractor. This deserves a detailed explanation.

The fundamental mistake made by Aneurin Bevan in 1948 and not remedied by NHS Management, was to allow the GPs to be self-employed. And worse still, for every doctor to own the practice, like many old-fashioned London city firms of solicitors, accountants, finance, insurance etc. All GPs became owners, possessing unique powers to pass on this ownership to anyone they liked, imparting on them the same rights in perpetuity. Initially, the GPs offered partnerships to colleagues, with a share of the practice income, becoming full partners after several years as agreed. As time progressed, transferable ownership of a GP practice has created massive problems.

You may be surprised to know that the entire system of the General Practices providing Primary Care to 56.5 million people in England is owned by 17,000 GP Partners. (NHS Digital)

Everyone in England is registered as a 'patient' with one of these doctors, practicing singly or in big partnerships, generating the income per GP, based on the number of people registered. The number of all GPs in England to include salaried doctors, trainee registrars and locums is 35,273. (NHS Digital)

These 17,000 GPs have a contract with the NHS to offer all the primary care services to the people of England and employ the rest of the 18,000 GP workforce. They are called GP contractors. This has created a culture of haves and have-nots, employers and employees. Apart from the good fortune to be holders of GP contractor status and older, they do not have any special qualifications or merit. They are called GP contractors but do not fit in with the criterion and definition of a 'contractor'.

By definition: "a contractor is a person or company that works on a contractual basis, negotiating deals with different clients to work on specific jobs or projects. Contactors are not employees and do not carry out regular work for a single employee. Contractors are therefore considered freelancers." (citrushr.com)

'Contractors are professionals who provide skills or services to companies for a set period. They may be contracted for a set number of hours, a certain time frame or duration of a project. They are not employees and can work on one or multiple contracts at a time.' (chas.co.uk)

The GP contractors have been given unprecedented power. They are the owners of the general practice in England. A registrar GP in training commented:
"Sadly, unknown to the public, the current system of the General Practice is a 'cartel' of the GP contractors. They are responsible for the recruitment of all new GPs and not the NHS. They set the terms and conditions of work and payment structure and often, offer them the job of a non-profit sharing salaried GP."

My research confirmed that the *GP contractors*, dictate the location of the practices, opening of new surgeries/health centres, closure of the practices, hiring and firing of all staff including other GPs and NOT the NHS. Ninety-nine practices closed in 2019, forcing nearly 350,000 people to move to a new surgery. (GPs magazine, Pulse)

This has inevitably resulted in greater number of GPs in more affluent areas. For example:

Northwest London	54 GPs /100,000 people
Kent, Surrey, Sussex	59 GPs /100,000 people
Wessex	61 GPs /100,000 people
South West	69 GPs /100,000 people
(Nuffield Trust)	

This disparity in the number of GPs in different parts of the country demonstrates that the NHS is NOT in control of

General Practice; GP-contractors and the private companies are.

On a different matter, a young salaried partner confided: "The General Practice is now a luxury lifestyle for most of the GP contractors, who on average do no more than four to six sessions a week whilst we the junior salaried doctors do up to ten sessions a week and see more than two to three times the number of patients and earn half or less. Cynically this could be described as "slave labour" and is rife in the English General Practice."

The overwhelming conclusion of my research is that most of the GP contractors spend more time in management activities, to maximise the practice profit and their take home money, than seeing patients.

Here's the story of an ex-hospital doctor, now a GP: "I spent six years in NHS hospitals, with no security of a job at the next level, took my turn for the night duties, weekends and relentless pressures to study and pass the post graduate exams. My friends who had joined General Practice as a contractor had bought nice homes, with kids in the local schools, whilst my wife and I lived in a modest two-bed rented apartment, not knowing where my next job would take me to and what school next for our daughter.

After discussion with my wife, I decided that becoming a GP contractor rather than waiting for another eight years to become a consultant was the best option. And oh boy, I found the General Practice to be heaven. No night duties, all weekends free, working, just office hours. Wow, I had to pinch myself to believe it. Within a few months we bought a nice four-bed detached house. Our daughter is in a good and permanent school. And yes, I am making the same amount of money being a GP contractor as a hospital consultant, without waiting another six to eight years."

Chapter Two

The GP contractors and the private companies who own the General Practice in England enjoy and celebrate Sutton's law. Willie Sutton, when, questioned why he robs banks, replied, "because that's where the money is".

Contrary to the traditions and practices of every Public Sector Service in England, the General Practice is now a money-making machine for GP contractors and private companies.

A thorough investigation into every Public Service Sector, does not reveal any profit generation activity, by the staff or the outside private companies. By very definition, the Public Sector is funded by the taxpayers and not subject to market forces and financial manipulations. What seemed an innocent loophole that allowed GPs to be self-employed, has now been turned into a money-making machine.

A Chartered Accountant said:
"In principle, a plumber has no possibility of self-employment status, if he works full-time for one employer and 98-99% of his total income is generated from that one employer. If such a scenario is discovered, both the employer and the employee would be harshly treated by HMRC for evading the tax liabilities. The arrangements by which a GP can be self-employed, drawing an income and additional perks based on the number of patients on her list, from one employer, the NHS, is beyond my comprehension and surely is caught under HMRC IR35 rules"

Bevan's General Practice of 1948 has been changed from a Patient-Centred Service to a Money Making/ For Profit Service. GP contractors and private companies are grabbing money from the taxpayers, thanks to the mindless reforms of the NHS management. Here is a brief introduction to the money-making activities within the General Practice.

Lucky to gain full partnerships, some of the GP contractors are entrepreneurs who've bought up the smaller, financially weaker practices. These doctors-turned-businessmen, delegate their patient consultation sessions to the non-profit sharing Salaried GPs by employing them at lesser salaries. Many have been known to boast, cynically: "The smaller the number of patients I see, the richer I get".

The rewards for exploiting a Public Service, funded by the taxpayers, to make personal profits, without improving any service to the patients are outrageous and baffling.

One GP earned	£600,000 - £700,000 pensionable pay.
Another received	£500,000 - £600,000.
14 were paid	£300,000 - £400,000.
with 146 earning	£200,000 - £300,000.
Nearly 5,500 earned	£100,000 - £200,000.

(PA Press Association, Nick Mc Dermott, The Sun)

There is no suggestion that every GP Contractor makes this money.

I now turn to private companies offering instant appointments (face-to-face, telephone, video): The well-publicised information of long waits to get GP appointments, has started a 'gold rush' by investors, to create brand new companies. Their promise? "There is no need to wait to see a GP, pay us and we we'll provide you with an instant appointment." The avalanche has created numerous regional and national companies.

Here are a few:

Doctaly: the company enables people to book a convenient, face-to-face consultation with an NHS GP on a private fee-paying basis. They compare themselves to the taxi company Uber (who incidentally lost the court case to maintain their taxi drivers as self-employed). The charge is £49.99 for a face-to-face consultation and £25 for a video consultation. The company is currently operating in Manchester, the West Midlands, Kent, Surrey, and Scotland. They plan to extend their services to 10,000 practices nationally and have signed deals with 35 GP practices, at the time of writing. The company has attracted 1134 private UK investors from Crowdcube and operates as BDM Medical Ltd. Company no 09305354.

Zoom Doc: in addition to providing online, video and telephone consultations, the company states, "We come to your home, hotel, office, we have a growing team of GPs that are available for home visiting consultations in minutes." The company claims to have GP and hospital partners, hotel and tourism partners, pharmacy partners and insurance partners. The investors are E-man Asset Management Ltd, Halkan Properties Ltd., Seeders Ltd and some private individuals.

GP DQ: 'GP Delivered Quickly' is a private service where patients can request a GP and track their progress through the GPDQ app, using a smartphone. Starting from London, expanding to Birmingham, the company claims that the service is now national. The cost for the private GP consultation is £49. The parent company of GPDQ is PDQ Technologies Ltd. Company no 09629824.

Medic Spot: provides patients with an online GP service through kiosks placed in pharmacies. You can walk in for a consultation without an appointment. The charge for a GP consultation is £39. The company is now located in 50 pharmacies nationally and claims to open in another 30 UK cities. Medic Spot Ltd. Company no 10089666.

Push Doctor: one of several companies offering digital/video consultations with a GP. They claim to have a network of 7,000 GMC reregistered GPs, who are available from 6am to 11pm,7 days a week, 365 days a year. The company has a monthly membership plus a consultation fee. Non-members can use the service for a fixed fee. Push Doctor claims to be the first video consultation provider, whereby any NHS GP can have real time access to NHS patients' records, using the company's digital platform. The three main investors are Oxford Capital Partners, Draper Espirit and Accelerated Development Venture (ADV), contributing close to £40 million (exact figure not available) Push DR Ltd. Company no 08624572.

The GP Service UK Ltd: claims to be open 365 days a year, 8am to 8pm; 95% prescriptions are processed by the company doctors, over 200 local walk-in centres, serving 6,000 pharmacies. Company doctors can access an electronic summary from the patient's records. Consultation £39 per doctor, prescription processing fee £7.49, fit notes free. Company no 09359853.

There are over 30 private companies reregistered with the Care Quality Commission providing instant GP appointments, operating locally, regionally and nationally. The big private hospital owners have also joined the gold rush including the Nuffield, BUPA, and BMI.

A female patient brought to my attention the following: "I wanted to consult my GP for a worrying personal problem.

I was offered a telephone appointment after 10 working days (two weeks) and was told that due to the pandemic, a face-to-face appointment was not available. I was able to secure a face-to-face appointment through a private company in the next two days. I was shocked to note that the GP who I consulted with is a full-time partner in the practice I am registered with. It's the same practice who couldn't even offer me a telephone appointment for two weeks. This is shockingly unfair and unjust. How could this be allowed to happen?"

I told her that my research shows that all the GPs, serving the private companies and offering instant appointments but unable to offer an NHS appointment for two weeks to their reregistered patents are fully paid NHS GPs, with six weeks holidays, gold-plated pension schemes and sick pay benefits! I am unable to repeat her telephone outbursts, in this PG rated work of non-fiction.

The NHS management has lost the plot relating to the General Practice in England. It is now the rule of the jungle, Darwin's law of survival of the fittest. The NHS GP says:
"No, I cannot offer you an appointment for two weeks from my NHS practice, but if you are prepared to pay me through a private company, yes, I am at your service now"

Several private companies are now offering General Practice Services on behalf of the NHS.

Babylon Healthcare Services Ltd: the company was the subject of Chapter 17 of my book "NHS is Not Working". I am providing you more in-depth details into the operations of this company because the Health Secretary at that time Matt Hancock publicly endorsed Babylon by declaring: "My GP is through the NHS on Babylon, it's brilliant".

Babylon's Ali Parsa was to commence a new era of the NHS Trust hospitals management as CEO of a private company, Circle Holding, a few years ago. He claimed that the private sector headed by him will show the nation, why the NHS had such a record of mismanagement and how he would change the way all the hospitals in England should be managed in future by the private sector.

He failed spectacularly and was forced to terminate the 10 year-contract of Hinchingbrooke Hospital after two years. The hospital trust was declared 'Inadequate overall' by the Care Quality Commission. Most damning, it was the first hospital trust that the watchdog had ever found to be inadequate in all areas. He resigned.

According to the Guardian, Ali Parsa was the sole beneficiary of this disastrous exercise and was paid £1.1 million. The same, Mr. Ali Parsa incorporated a company "Babylon Healthcare Services" in 2014.

Babylon's net worth in 2015 was £11,409. At that time, Ali Parsa's Babylon's website stated, "Babylon is home to the largest collection of scientists, mathematicians and engineers."

I have been unable to unveil the mystery of the company, headed by a person with a well-known history of corporate failure, allowed to start and own the taxpayer's public sector General Practice "GP at Hand".

Anyone can join Babylon's services and be promised a 'no-wait prompt GP appointment' through a mirage of remote telephone and video appointments. But you cannot be registered and offered a service, if you have any of the following existing medical conditions:

Pregnancy, adults with safeguarding needs, people with complex mental health conditions, people with complex physical, psychological/social needs, those with dementia, older people with conditions related to frailty, people requiring end of life care, parents of children who are on the 'at risk' register, people with learning disabilities, people with drug dependence.

In other words, Babylon's GP services are available only to the young and healthy whilst those with challenging medical conditions cannot join. According to a report published by GP Online, "of the 31,519 new patients who have signed up with "GP at Hand", over the last 12 months, 87% are aged between 20 to 39. Those who are over 65 now make up only 1%."

The refusal of Babylon, to provide General Practice services to people with pre-existing conditions can have serious existential threat to the NHS. Think of a situation, where 40% of the young and healthy people, move to companies like Babylon. The income of the practices would be reduced by 40% (GPs are paid per person and not for each appointment). However, the number of appointments by the rest of the 60 % of patients needing attention, would hardly decline. The practice would not be able to operate as a financially viable proposition and would go out of business.

Imagine now a long-term scenario, where there are no GPs available to look after those with challenging physical and mental conditions. Destabilisation of local health economy is a serious threat, as shown above. Hammersmith & Fulham CCG, where GP at Hand is based, now has a serious financial deficit.

The most worrying aspect is the support and endorsement by the Health Secretary at that time, Matt Hancock. The position of a Health Secretary who does not understand the fundamentals of the NHS General Practice, is untenable. He has since resigned, not for his inability to understand and embrace the workings of the NHS General Practice but 'embrace' of a different kind that you may have learned from the press and the TV.

The range of investors is worth noting: Swedish Investment Group AB Kinnevik, BXR group, Demis Hassabis and Mustafa Suleyman, Hoxton ventures, Sawiris, NNS Holdings, Vostok New Ventures, Saudi Arabia's Public Investment Fund, Munich Re's ERGO Fund etc.
Company no 09229684.Babylon Health Care Services was incorporated in 2014. Company No 09229684. Only one company director Mr. Ali Parsadoust

LIVI: This company from Sweden has created an online app to introduce digital GP services to the UK, in collaboration with existing GP surgeries. It appears that initially the GP consultations would be carried out by the GPs employed by LIVI. The company has been 'commissioned' to provide digital appointments to NICS (Northwest Surrey Integrated Care Services) which is GP Federation that brings together 38 GP practices caring for 380,000 patients. LIVI appears to be working for partnerships with Birmingham's Our Health Partnership, Northampton General Practice Alliance, Shropshire Alliance for Better Care and several more, details of which are not available at this stage.

In April 2020, Boots and LIVI formed a partnership to have a live video GP service in the stores of Boots. LIVI is a subsidiary of the Swedish Healthcare Group KRY, managed by Webbhalsa. Details about the investors is difficult to obtain. It appears that LIVI/KRY had four major investments of 20 million Euros and a further 53 million Euros from Index Ventures. It has not been possible to establish how much of it would go towards the UK General Practice. LIVI provides no information about its financial activities to the Companies House, as it is a Swedish company.

Integral Medical Holdings Ltd.: The company manages a network of 11 GP Practices and has a further seven contracts delivering, 'out of hours', Urgent Treatment Centres and Walk in Centres.

US Health Insurance Giant Centene: In 2001, two GPs started The Practice Group. The company would offer 100% purchase (or partial equity scheme) to the single hand GPs wanting early retirement and small practices and then employ the GP owners as salaried doctors. This model seemed to work, and the company had 16 contracts with GP surgeries. Further expansion took place through acquisition of other companies:
Chilvers McCrea. With over 30 surgeries
United Health UK. - 6 surgeries
Phoenix Primary Care Ltd - 12 surgeries.

The company was bought in 2016 by the US Fortune 500 company Centene Corporation. Centene brought together its two subsidies, The Practice Group and Simplify Health under one brand 'Operose Health'. Centene is now the owner of Operose Health and by taking over AT Medics, the company is currently operating 70 GP surgeries in England.

Virgin Care Ltd: One of the enterprises of the goateed, self-publicist, UK entrepreneur, Richard Branson, whose NHS targeted company is said to have paid no tax since 2010. At present, Virgin operates 30 Primary Care services, including 19 GP surgeries.

Modality Partnership: an example of a super partnership of 48 surgeries, apparently led by twelve 'leader GPs', operating with 54 full-time and 201 part-time GPs. The company refused to provide information on the actual take away annual income of the 'twelve leaders', nor the number of patients consulted in each session.

The NHS General Practice is in a mess. There is a mushrooming of GP practices, from a single hand GP to small group practices, GP federations, GP super partnerships, private companies and now the brainchild of NHS England, the Primary Care Networks. National and international investors see the General Practice as a golden opportunity to make money.

Politicians, academics and some left-wing activists have been worrying and protesting about the threat of 'the NHS General Practice Privatisation'. The fact is that the NHS General Practice in England is a commercial enterprise, run for profit by the GP contractors and the private companies.

Chapter Three

Here are two astonishing discoveries about the General Practice which took me weeks to stumble upon, and that you may find amusing or scandalous.

Medical science has evolved to a bewildering series of new techniques of diagnosis, treatment, and life-changing operative techniques. There are more than 60 disease-related specialities in England, each speciality may have several sub specialities, practiced from the modern hospitals by the "super specialists". All these highly complex fields of medicines can only be delivered from hospitals equipped with sophisticated diagnostic facilities and operating theatres.

The speciality of the simple, ancient, noble, General Practice has not changed since the inception of the NHS in 1948, and for that matter even 100 years before.

All that a GP needs to perform his duties is a consulting room with a hand wash sink, an examination couch, a doctor's chair, a desk for a computer and two chairs for the patients, all of which are housed in an eight-square-metre room. The equipment required can be accommodated on a small table, with room to spare; the proverbial stethoscope, instruments to check blood pressure, examine eyes, ears, and throat, and oh, gloves. Believe it or not, that's it.

You could be awed to see a grand Health Centre, with dozens of dedicated car parking spaces for the staff. The bulk of the impressive building is occupied by an army of receptionists, nurses, paramedics, managers, phlebologists, podiatrists, all appearing to help GP contractors, salaried doctors, and locums.

But are any extra room facilities essential for the GP to consult a patient? No. The GP does not need to have nurses and paramedics in the same building to go about their work.

In fact, there's no evidence that the standards of GP consultations are better from the grand Health Centres than from the modest small old surgery buildings.

The simplicity of the General Practice has become overly complicated, and ambiguity and confusion now overwhelm the reality. Sir Simon Stevens, the CEO of NHS England, ex US health Insurance supremo, having failed to make any impact on any aspect of the General Practice for four years, has decided on a 10-year plan. This period is long enough for the CEO not to be held accountable and retire with a gold-plated pension, hopefully to the house of lords. Clever.

Sir Simon Stevens has left as the CEO of NHS England at the end of July 2021 and has been made a peer. (Sky News)

As a part of the 10-year plan, all the GP Practices no matter what their size, must now join one of the 1250 PCN's (Primary Care Networks). An analyst commented that without a degree in business administration, it may be difficult to comprehend the new management structure involving General Practice.

"Primary Care Networks will be focussed on service delivery, rather than on the planning and funding of services, responsibility for which will remain with commissioners and are expected to be the building blocks around which integrated systems are built. The ambition is that Primary Care Networks will be the mechanism by which primary care representation is made stronger in integrated care systems, with the accountable clinical directors from each network being the link between general practice and the wider system."

There is no mention of the possibility of anyone waiting less than two weeks to get a GP appointment or being able to have a face-to-face consultation with a GP over the weekend or after 6 pm.

Here's how the taxpayer's money is going to fund the General Practice.

"The main funding for PCN's (Primary Care Networks) comes in the form of DES, direct enhanced services payment. Networks also receive payments from Investment and Impact Fund, a financial scheme like the Quality and Outcomes Framework that rewards networks for performance. The additional income would be generated by

- PCN Funding
- Clinical director contribution
- Additional Roles Reimbursement Scheme Payments
- Care Home Premiums
- PCN support payment
- Extended hour access payments
- Investment and Impact Fund
- Network Participation Payment (NHS England)

Once it has been clarified that unlike the hospital super-specialists, requiring sophisticated and ever-changing equipment, all that a GP needs to consult is an 8 square meter room and nothing else, understanding of the proposed changes would be easier.

Having examined Think Tank research (King's Fund, Health Foundation, Nuffield Trust) no firm conclusions have been drawn and sadly no red signals waved on the deteriorating waiting to access a GP appointment, nor the extraordinary delegation of the practice patients care to the NHS 111 *(Chapter six)* and worse of all to the A&E departments.

The obstacles to reform are massive and warrant repeating.

1. Declining number of GPs over the last two decades, with a growing population.
2. Change of the General Practice model from a 24/7 essential public service to a profit-making commercial enterprise, operating Mon to Fridays; 8am -6pm.
3. A guaranteed income to every GP practice based on the number of patients registered with the GP contractors, without any accountability or adverse consequences for making them wait for 2 weeks to get an appointment.
4. The unfortunate mindset of every GP is that the General Practice is the same as a solicitor's or accountants' practice, with no night duties, no weekend work. Full time GPs offer 9 sessions a week to see patients; morning and evening, the fifth day is a half day. This is in total contradiction to the medical profession's work ethics where the hospital colleagues do regular night duties and weekend work. Most GP contractors appear to offer 4-6 sessions a week in which they see patients, spending the remaining time in management activities.

My instinct told me that there was something missing. The words of Paul Krugman the Nobel Prize winning Economist, repeatedly echoed in my mind, 'Productivity isn't everything, but in the long term, it is almost everything.'

One evening, tired and frustrated, I dug into the piles of statistical information and made two discoveries.

First, the General Practice in England is being run by GPs, 75.7% of whom work part-time only. The following are the working hours of all Qualified Permanent GPs In England (excluding locums and trainee registrars).

PART TIME 15 hours or less   8.2%

PART TIME greater than 15 hours
but less than 37.5 hours   67.5 %

FULL TIME 37.5 hours or more   24.3%
(NHS Digital)

Second, the Qualified Permanent GPs in England, stop working as they age (excluding locums and trainee registrars).

Number of doctors in General Practice, age 30 to 44 years = 55.2% of the existing workforce

Number of doctors in General Practice, age 45 to 54 years = 25.06% of the existing workforce

Number of doctors in General Practice, age 55 to 59 years = 10.58% of the existing workforce

Number of doctors in General Practice, age 60 to 64 years = 4.58 % of the existing workforce

Number of doctors in General Practice, age 65 and over = 3.17% of the existing workforce

Unknown
= Approximate 1 % of the existing workforce

The mysteriously disappearing numbers of Qualified Permanent GPs in England, as they age is worth noting:

Between ages of 45 - 54 the GPs number is reduced by 45.39% from the age group 30 - 44 years

Between ages of 55 - 59 the GPs number is reduced by 42.61% from the age group 45 - 54 years

Between ages of 60 - 64 the GP number is reduced by 43.28% from the age group 55 - 59 years

At 65 and over, the GP number is reduced by 69.21% from the age group 60 - 64 years
(NHS Digital)

The cataclysm of the part time deployment of the GPs by the self-employed GP contractors, points to a management disarray, never witnessed in any private, public, or voluntary sector before. Nor is it possible to explain the declining number of the GPs who from the age of 45 decide to stop working for the NHS, or is it? One explanation might be to make lucrative sums by working for the private GP companies.

The sole reason for most of the ills of the General Practice is the self-employed status of the GP contractors. My biggest and game changing recommendation, in one paragraph, is as follows:
"The toxic system of self-employment status of the GPs should be abolished, as they no longer offer 24/7 service, which was the main criterion of giving them the self-employment status at the inception of the NHS in 1948. Every GP would be paid a salary, based on the number of appointment sessions offered in a week and no longer on the number of persons registered in the name of a GP contractor in a practice. Steps would be taken to significantly increase the number of 'patient consultation sessions' to assure same-day or

next-day appointments, availability after 6 pm and the weekends". (Details in following chapters.)

All hospital doctors are paid a salary, same as employees of other public services. If the self-employment/profit generating system of the General Practice were to be adapted by the Police, Ambulance, Fire, and Hospitals, we would have no Public Service in England.

Fyodor Dostoyevsky famously stated, 'Man is a creature that can get accustomed to anything.' Those running The NHS Management agree that people in England should get accustomed to the General Practice as it is.

In the early 20th century, business owners believed that "the businesses are run for the benefit of the owners.' In the mid and late 20th century, the business owners realised that in reality 'the businesses are run for the benefit of the customers."

Sadly, the General Practice in England is conducted for the benefit of the employees and not for the benefit of the people needing medical attention.

Imagine, police stations run by self-employed senior police officers, deciding where to locate, hiring the new police officers at half their own take home pay, working 8am to 6 pm, strictly Monday to Friday and asking the Govt. to cover crimes (burglary, grievously body harm, rape and similar) after 6pm and over the weekends through 'out of hours services' as they have decided to opt out. This is how the General Practice is run in England!

Chapter Four

How the people of England and the treasury would benefit if the self-employed status of the 17,000 or so GP contractors, employing 18,000 doctors and over 100,000 staff, were abolished. The return of the family doctor.

The single one act to abolish the self-employed status of the GPs would allow the NHS to take control and eliminate the historical hierarchical ownership of a practice passed on for decades from one GP contractor to the next. All GPs would be employed by the NHS and paid a salary by the NHS, empowering the majority to be independent of the shackles and demands of the GP contractors and private companies. Every aspect of the General Practice infrastructure would be standardised nationally.

Current consultation times: ostensibly, these are between 8am to 6pm, Monday to Friday, but the actual consultation times all over England vary greatly. The average national and acknowledged time given to each GP appointment is ten minutes, with 18 persons seen in each three-hour session. A full-time GP is supposed to offer five morning and four evening sessions. This would mean 162 persons seen face-to-face in a five-day week. Sessions rarely end after 6pm.

The recommended new consultation times:
Mornings: 9.30 -12.30.   Five weekdays
Afternoon/Evenings   4pm – 7pm   Four weekdays

The proposed times have advantages for patients, especially those who work away from the home and would be able to secure appointments between 6pm to 7pm without taking time off. These consultation hours should be national, with no flexibility to change to suit the individual needs of any GPs.

Every GP should work a certain number of evening sessions, night duties and weekends, as do over 100,000 of their hospital colleagues. The General Practice must offer face-to-face consultation service for non-routine medical problems after 6 pm and over the weekends, as is customary in every affluent country in the world.

Proposed GP 'after hours' consultation sessions:
- 6pm to 9 pm
- 9pm to 12 am
- 12 am to 8 am

Proposed GP consultation sessions, Saturdays and Sundays:
- 11am to 2 pm, 3pm to 6pm

In Chapter Five, I'll provide details of how many of these after hour and weekend sessions, each GP should offer over a 12-month period and it's actually not many.

As if waiting for an appointment for two weeks wasn't bad enough, some of the stories I've heard about some patients dealing with receptionists are mind blowing. One woman told me:

"It took me two hours for two mornings and one over two evenings on the telephone to get through to the practice receptionist; the phone was engaged all the time. I was handed over an appointment after 11 working days. On attending my appointment, I was astonished to see that in the main reception, a screen which showed:

Inbound calls:	367
Inbound answered:	282
Inbound abandoned:	85
Max waiting time:	22 minutes.

It appears there is no stone unturned to deter people from seeking medical help from the first and only contact with the medical profession. A few years ago, there was a furious backlash from the media about the GP receptionists training to be 'care navigators', with a standard question they were required to ask: "Why do you want to see the GP?"

I propose that the introduction of an online appointments system should replace the telephone system. It is of prime importance to terminate the telephone appointment system. Instead, two online appointment portal systems could be introduced, covering all GPs currently in a practice and every GP in an area within 10-15 miles radius. The Monday to Friday online appointments portal system would replace the existing antiquated telephone method. The out of hours and weekend online appointments system would replace the telephone call centre NHS 111.

Processes can be put in place to ensure that the 'out of hours and weekend services' are for genuine semi-urgent or urgent medical problems and not used to substitute the routine matters that could have been dealt with before 7pm and on weekdays. Several telephone lines would be made available to those with no access to the internet or inability to use it.

Every one of us in England is registered with a GP practice. The increasing profit-focussed infrastructure has resulted in GP contractors seeing fewer patients by employing salaried doctors, locums, advance nurse practitioners, physician associates at a lower salary. The result is that the traditional family doctor has all but disappeared.

"Almost half of primary care patients can no longer name a single GP at their own surgery, a poll has revealed. Medics say the findings suggest the days of having a dedicated family doctor are over. Just one in three see the same doctor every time, a third see two different GPs a year and a fifth see three." (practicebusiness.co.uk)

The same publication states that research shows that "the elderly patients who see the same GP each time are less likely to need hospital treatment".

In the new proposed structure, the total number of 56.5 million people in England (including children) would be divided by the number of all practitioners; to exclude trainee registrars and locums. Every GP would be given responsibility to look after a certain nominated number of people, making sure that there is an equal and fair number of people allocated to each doctor, based on age and gender. Keeping in mind my research that 75% of the GPs, work part-time, an individual could have more than one nominated GP.

What a great feeling to know that you and I and everyone else would have one or two nominated family doctors, responsible for our health and welfare. This is likely to give the GPs greater job satisfaction with personal ownership and responsibility to the nominated people under their stewardship.

Let us now examine the reformed management infra-structure of a GP practice. Years of subsidies by the NHS to the GP Practices have resulted in a robust management structure within each practice. Whereas the focus of all management activities by the GP contractors is to maximise personal profit, all activities of the practice are run, managed, and supervised by the practice manager, practice nurses, receptionists, and the other miscellaneous staff.

You may be interested to know that GPs have no participation in ante natal & post-natal care, cervical smears, children's vaccinations, flu vaccination, travel vaccination. The practice nurses operate, asthma, hypertension, diabetes, weight management and stop smoking clinics.

The abolition of self-employed status will have no impact on the provision of day-to-day routine consultations to the people. The practice manager would have a greater input into the practice management by maximising the uptake of cervical smears and the various immunisations. The disease management clinics would continue to be run by the practice nurses. The absurd system whereby the GP contractors, who do not have the slightest input to meet certain income generating targets, would end, saving a significant amount of money.

Currently all the running expense of every GP Practice in England, is borne by the NHS. The NHS makes the payment for rent/mortgage of the premises to the GP Practices, which then transfer this amount received to the owners, landlords or the mortgage company. The salaries of all practice staff, including receptionists, telephonists, cleaners, nurses and practice managers (except the salaried GPs) are paid by the NHS to the Practices. This sum is then paid by the practices to every member of the staff as salaries!

With the new arrangement, the NHS would make all payments directly to those concerned and eliminate the tedious arrangements and the profit-making GP contractors and the private companies, acting as middlemen.

The only expenses not paid by the NHS are rates, utility bills, postage and stationery. These overheads are paid from the very lucrative profits achieved by the GP Contractors and the private companies. All such payments would be paid directly by the NHS to achieve significant overall savings. Such financial arrangements are the normal practice. The treasury pays overheads of all the public service institutions like schools, hospitals, fire, ambulance, police etc.

Chapter Five

Even Sherlock Holmes might have struggled to solve the perplexing mystery of the inequality in GPs' take-home salary, it ranges from £45,000 to £700,000 a year.

In most private and public service, the staff salaries have a definite structure, based on the academic qualifications, experience and longevity of service. The NHS is no different. There are nine bands, from Band one to Band nine and Band eight is split into A, B, C, D.

Hospital doctors have a different structure of salaries starting from House Officer to Consultant. A speciality registrar, still in training after six years of graduation, can languish at a salary ranging from £42,969 to £51,069 (nhsemployers.org).

From NHS England:
The estimated average income before tax of GPs:
£98,000 when contractor and salaried GPs are combined.
When split:
£117,300, for contractor GPs
£60,600, for salaried GPs

GP Practices are required to publish their GPs' Net Earnings on their websites. I decided to test the marketplace by having this information from two very large GP Practices.

GP Net earnings before tax and national insurance:
Babylon GP at Hand: £83,420.83 for fifty-three part-time GPs (At the time of writing, the information on their website was three years old, with no updates, contrary to the guidelines.)

Modality Partnership: £66,200 for 54 full-time and 201 part-time GPs. Modality refused to provide information about the GP net earnings of its 12 GP contractors/leaders.

I decided to search for several GP practices in one city. Here are the rather astonishing results, which I've grouped from lower to higher wages.

Average GP Net Earnings, before tax and NI, as shown on the twenty randomly chosen websites of one city:

£44,870

£52, 969	£53,574	£55,684	£56,937
£57,588,	£58,606		
£62,468	£66,648	£68,694	
£71,730	£73,025	£79,498	
£81,108	£88,627	£88,902	
£98,904	£98,876		

£120,342

£240,084

I mentioned in Chapter Two that "One GP earned £600,000 to £700,000 in pensionable pay, another got £500,000 to £600,000, several earning £200,000 to £400,000."

To be truthful, I find this kind of inequality, disparity and irregularity in the GP pay structure disquieting. In chapter three, I've pointed out that 75 % of doctors in the General Practice work part-time but I also found that the part-timers on average work two days (out of five, the full-timers do). So, the unanswered question:

What could be the explanation for one GP taking home just £44,870 and another, in the same city, 5.4 times more at £240,084?
The UK Prime Minister salary, for comparison, is £161,401.

Please note, the stated declaration by NHS England of GPs' net earnings does not relate to any of the figures that I have researched. You will agree that the salaries of the GPs, once the self-employed status of the GP contractors is terminated, must be based on principles of fairness and justice and in keeping with the work ethics and remuneration status of their hospital colleagues.

To recap, a full time GP offers 9 consultation sessions to the people in one week; five in the morning, four in the afternoon, Monday to Friday, 8am to 6 pm. Traditionally one day out of five, there are no afternoon sessions. Eighteen appointments are offered in one session, e.g., 162 persons in one week. No work after 6pm, no weekend work.

Here is my recommendation. In chapter four, my most important recommendation was to bring the working practices of the GPs in line with their hospital colleagues and for every GP, part-time, full-time, trainee registrar to do the following 'after hours sessions' over a 12-month period

Every GP to work, over a period of 12 months (To exclude locums but include registrars)

On weekdays:

6 pm to 9 pm	Six Sessions per year
9 pm to 12 midnight	Six Sessions per year
12 midnight to 8 am	Two Sessions per year

Saturdays and Sundays:
11am to 2 pm and 3 pm to 6 pm - just 6 weekends, spread out over the year.

To put things in perspective, GPs would work on just six weekends in a 12-month period: two three-hour consultation sessions on Saturdays, and the same on Sundays. Please note, this weekend working does not include working at night. This is unlike their hospital colleagues, who are present or on call for the entire period, from Friday afternoon to Monday morning including nights.

The "after hours sessions" to include only two-night duties for the entire 12-month period would be considered a mini holiday by the hospital doctors! The GPs would be given no choice to opt out of these new hours.

My recommended salary at the commencement of a new GP appointment is £70,000, as Band One. This should attract more doctors to join General Practice.

Recent data from HMRC shows that the median average pre-tax income is around £22,400. An income of £70,000 a year would put a new GP in the top five per cent of all UK earners" (The Independent Newspaper)

As stated earlier, all the new GP recruitments would be made by the NHS management, in areas where more GPs are needed (Chapter One).

All GPs would have the same employed status and GP Contractors would no longer exist!

The proposed salary structure would be as follows for those working full time and pro-rata for part time GPs:

Band One	Service 1 - 5 years	£70,000
Band Two	Service 6-10 years	£80,000
Band Three	Service 11-16 years	£90,000
Band Four	Service over 16 years	£100,000

There would also be great opportunities for GPs to enhance their NHS salary by offering additional sessions to patients.

Every GP would be allowed to offer more sessions and the following is a list of 'bonuses' for those wanting to do additional sessions to the statutory work:

Weekends:	£800
6pm – 9pm	£300
9pm -12 midnight	£400
12 midnight -8am	£800

Please imagine a scenario: A GP decides to offer in addition:
One evening session 6pm - 9pm, for 40 weeks, would earn an extra £12,000 annually.
One evening session 9pm - 12pm for ten weeks would earn an extra £4,000 annually.
Four weekend sessions would earn an extra £3,200 annually.
Two-night duty sessions would earn an extra £1,600 annually.

A potential to earn £20,800 extra, in total per year more.

My salary recommendations are far superior for the GPs than their hospital colleagues, several of whom are still being trained, still studying, still desperate to pass post graduate exams, still working nights, still working weekends, still without their own residence, still renting after 8 - 12 years service, before getting the job of a consultant.

Chapter Six

Nowhere on planet earth, except in England, are an entire population of a rich country denied 'face-to-face' GP consultations after 6 pm or at the weekends. Yet, shockingly, for 110 hours every week, the call centre NHS 111 provides treatment by telephone only.

The inability of NHS management, to find a solution to any problem is heart-stopping. While claiming a high satisfaction level of the public with the General Practice, the depressing inability of those in need to see a GP was becoming disturbing to those at the helm of the NHS management. The solution came in the form of creating a wholly inadequate parallel GP universe called NHS 111.

An anonymous NHS manager is known to have said: "We have created the NHS 111, available 24/7 because we know that those in need are unable to get a GP appointment, even on weekdays between 8am to 6 pm. Surely, something is better than nothing."

The most damning fact about the General Practice in England is that the GP you are registered with provides just 50 hours a week of medical attention, out of 168 hours. Your first contact for seeking medical attention during the remaining 118 hours is to talk on the telephone to a 'Health Adviser' of the NHS 111, who will decide what your best course of treatment is.

You'd think that those looking after the primary care needs of the nation as the 'first contact' in the NHS 111, must be highly trained and qualified people. Just read the advertisement to hire NHS 111 respondents:

"You must be 18, have the right to work in the UK, be committed to excellence to our patients, caring and understanding, good communications skills, commitment to quality. You will need to be able to commit to a six-week programme to become fully trained, which will be fully paid." (jobs.nhs.uk)

Please note that no background, qualification, or experience relating to care, nursing or medical matters is required. As long as you are over 18 and are committed to 6 weeks training, you can now go ahead and join the NHS111. The six weeks training has been a favourite joke of the media and here is one report:
"Shocking footage inside NHS 111 training centre shows tutors having their eyebrows threaded before giving trainees the answers for exams for life-or-death jobs. At the end of the course, it was alleged that the struggling trainees were given answers in the medical exam, enabling "utterly incompetent people" to qualify as "Health Advisers"
(Exclusive report by Jake Wallis Simons, Associate Global Editor for the Mail online)

You can well imagine the stress experienced by the unqualified staff, dealing with medical problems on the telephone and trying to find the best solution, from a scripted questionnaire. Psychologically, for the poor Health Advisers, it must feel like the "Charge of the Light Brigade" daily.

Another report:
"A senior call adviser at the scandal-hit NHS 111 centre has described a "terrifying" night shift when she was left in charge of the well-being of 400,000 people, despite having no medical qualification and no support from a nurse or a paramedic. (Independent.co.uk)

The outcomes of the chaotic telephone call handling service are predictable.

"Before Covid-19, NHS 111 had already been linked to safety failings, resulting in over 20 deaths. Horror stories include the death of two-year-old Myla Deviren, misdiagnosed with a stomach bug. Too many patients are being referred unnecessarily to already overstretched A&E, making it harder for critically ill patients to be seen." (MP Kate Osamore)

The stories of the incompetent handling of critical matters by 111, leading to tragic consequences are numerous and heart-breaking, such as this report:
"Mother tells how her son, four, died after "rude and abrupt" NHS 111 operator failed to spot that his rash and shortness of breath meant he was dangerously ill (dailymail.co.uk.)

And then there's the intolerable pressure put on the A&E departments by the NHS 111 Health Advisers telling people to go to A&E.

"Of all the calls received by the NHS 111, 22.5% were directed to go to the A&E, 12.5 % were referred to the Ambulance Service. 10% were recommended to go to their GP" (NHS England)

It appears that a significant number of people don't bother to contact 111 and head to A&E anyway. One woman told me: "I have taken advice from Jeremy Hunt (ex-Health Secretary), who famously said that he takes his kids to the A&E. Better to be seen and get treatment from a doctor face to face, even waiting for 6 hours, than the dubious telephone advice from NHS 111."

"A survey carried out after in the wake of a damming NHS 111 report into the death of one-year-old William Mead, found that

78% of mothers would go straight to the A&E rather than call NHS 111, if their child is sick."
(survey - Net Mums.)

These findings paint a bleak picture of the NHS 111 service. 84% of the reviews on 'Trust Pilot' rate NHS 111, as bad or poor.

NHS England has made available a list of 68, NHS 111 Centres operating throughout England following a Freedom of Information request. 75% of the NHS 111 call centres are provided and managed by 'not for profit' and social enterprises. The rest are run by private companies making good profit. To give an example:

Care UK	10 centres	
Vocare	3 centres	Turnover £ 60,227,874
Devon Doctors	3 centres	Turnover £ 36,610,090
Nedvivo Group	1 centre	Turnover £21,844,629

Care UK is a massive company, owns 110 care homes, domiciliary services, 60 NHS Primary care services, NHS 111 service etc. Owned by the private equity firm Bridgepoint Capital, it was not possible to find out the cost to the NHS of operating it's 10, NHS 111 centres.

Director's remuneration of the Devon Doctors was £826,321 and that of Nedvivo Group £457,932, according to the latest figures available.

Everyone in England who's had the shortest encounter with the NHS 111 is dismayed or openly disgusted. The common question being asked repeatedly was, 'is there no alternative to the call centre telephone treatment? Is it not possible for a GP to provide a face-to-face consultation instead?

Why isn't it possible? I decided to investigate.

Between December 2015 and December 2020, the average number of daily calls, the NHS 111 received averaged around 57,000 (NHS England)

If the NHS 111, dealing with 57,000 telephone calls in 24 hours, is replaced by face-to-face consultation by GPs, how could it work? Let us do some calculations.

The number of all qualified GPs to exclude the locums but include the qualified registrars, receiving training to be a GP is 33,982. (NHS Digital)

57,000 calls, divided by 33,982 GPs = 1.67 per GP per day,

My calculations, based on the number of all qualified GPs in England show that if the NHS 111 were to be abolished overnight, one GP needs to offer face-to-face consultation and treatment to a maximum of two patients in 24 hours (1.67).

The Healthcare Safety Investigation Branch (HSIB) has launched an investigation into the failings by the NHS 111 telephone advice service, which may have cost the lives of people with Covid-19. The Covid-19 Bereaved Families for Justice Group believes that several hundred of its members had a relative die after calling NHS 111 and being told that they should stay at home.

Ten nurses who worked for the NHS 111 Covid-19 Clinical Assessment Service have described it as shambolic and lacking in adequate training and safeguards. The former CCAS nurses came forward to talk about their experiences after it was revealed that an audit had found 60% of calls to patients by allied healthcare professionals had not been safe.
(The Guardian)

To delegate 70% responsibility of looking after the General Practice needs of people in England to the call centre NHS 111, forcing people registered with a GP to receive treatment by telephone only, must be considered as one of the most catastrophic decisions ever made in the history of healthcare provision, by any country in the world.

The NHS 111 has no place in the provision of Primary Care and must be scrapped as quickly as possible. I hope to provide a credible alternative solution in chapters that follows.

Chapter Seven

NHS England, academics of the Royal college of General Practitioners, advocates of the British Medical Association, stars of the three health-related think tanks, the politicians; all agree that the shortage of GPs is one of the major problems facing the General Practice in England. Amazingly, no one knows the number of GPs the General Practice is short of. My breakthrough numerical discovery has rocked me.

The NHS England has successfully convinced everyone that the General Practice is as good as anywhere else in a rich country and that the minor problems are due to a shortage of GPs, an increase in population and, above all, limited availability of funds. In other words, if the number of GPs could be increased, all the problems would be solved. This theory of GP shortages as the cause of all evils in NHS General Practice is now universally accepted.

"If services are to meet demand, another 5,000 full time GPs will be needed by 2020." (NHS England, Forward View)

This number of additional GPs has not been achieved.

"Our recent joint report with the Health Foundation and the King's Fund suggested the shortfall in GPs could grow by around 4,500 full-time equivalents in five years unless urgent action is taken" (Billy Palmer, Nuffield Trust)

The above statement by the three 'Giant Think Tanks' appears to suggest that the current number of GPs is satisfactory unless action is taken to keep up with the possible future shortage of numbers. A further declaration confirms:

'Our forecast that the shortfall in GPs would triple from 2,500 in 2019 to 7,000 by 2023-24 has not changed.' (Researcher Beccy Baird, King's Fund)

The 'GPs shortage numbers game' is an interesting political hobby too:

'The NHS needs 9,000 more GPs to deliver safe care, unions warn. The conservatives have promised 6,000 more GPs, Labour has promised 5,000 extra and the Liberal Democrats have promised to end the GP shortages in 5 years.' (Nick Bostock, gponline.com)

How many more GPs?

"The latest estimates from the Royal College of General Practitioners members" surveys and data suggest that the UK needs an extra 8,000 more GPs." (bhf.org.uk)

It is surprising that learned academics, GP leaders and most importantly, NHS England talk about GP shortages, without identifying the accurate numbers required. And without providing any evidence to demonstrate that certain increased numbers would relieve the misery of millions of people unable to get prompt GP appointments and millions more whose bodies have the unfortunate habit of developing symptoms after 6 pm and over the weekends. '54.1 million patients waited over 2 weeks to get GP appointment between February 2019 and 2020.' (British Medical Association)

Nothing can be more basic in any organisation than identifying the optimal number of persons required to undertake the series of all the essential tasks. Not so with the NHS General Practice. With 75% of the NHS GPs working part time, trying to find out the optimal numbers is complex. The demand for more GPs by the various institutions ranging from 5,000 to 9,000 is an assumption.

What we need to find out is the number of GP appointments required in order to provide face-to-face consultation to people in a 24-hour period, including after 6pm, through the nights and over the weekends.

In other words, in order to calculate the number of GPs required, we must find out, the number of GP appointments one person requires on average over a 12-month period. Let's consider the statistics.

"Nearly 38% of people in the European Union went to see their generalist medical practitioner once or twice in the twelve months prior to the survey. A quarter (25%) consulted their generalist medical practitioner 3-5 times, while nearly another quarter (24%) did not go to see a generalist medical practitioner. Denmark had the largest share of persons who saw their generalist medical practitioner 6 times or more (49%) during the previous 12 months, while France had 34% people going to doctor 3-5 times. Among the EU member states, there is a wide range in frequency, varying between 4.3 to 10. The highest number recorded seems to be Slovakia and Hungary- up to 10.9 consultations." (Eurostat, ec.europa.eu)

"Americans visit their doctor four times a year. People in Japan visit 13 times a year." (Niall McCarthy, Forbes.com)

Figures for England are different. The number of average GP consultations a year by one person is seven.
(Royal College of General Practitioners)

It is appropriate, to use the figures from the Royal College of General Practitioners, indicating the average number of visits per person to a GP in 12 months. You may be asking how correct is this figure of seven visits per person, per year? You may not have seen your GP all year, while your neighbour has seen them twice a month or more.

'For many outcomes, roughly 80% of the consequences come from 20% of the causes.' (Pareto's 80/20 principle)

It is possible that 20% of the population may create 80% of all appointments any day of the week over the 12-month period.

Calculation:
Total number of GP appointments required, based on an average of seven GP appointments per person per year, for the population in England of 56.5 million people:

56.5 million x 7 = 395,500,000 appointments.

The average number of GP appointments available to the people annually = 300 million (NHS England)

This shows a discrepancy of 95.5 million appointments, between what could be technically required and what the NHS England claims to offer. Unfortunately, the provision of a figure of 300 million GP appointments a year, does not take into consideration, a very crucial factor.

The Crucial Factor:
"45.4 % of all of GP appointments occurred with a non-GP healthcare professional. (British Medical Association)

This means that out of total number of 300 million annual appointments, the number of people who are seen by the General Practitioner doctors is 54.6% of the number:

300,000,000 x 54.6% = 163,800,000, annually. For the sake of simplicity, let us make it 164 million.

Let it be clear, the figures propagated by the NHS England of 300 million GP appointments offered to the people over one year are wrong. The number of appointments available to see a GP Doctor are only 164 million, the rest are with the Non-GP professionals within the GP practices. (136 million)

It has been shown previously that based on the average figure of seven consultations by every person in a year, the number of minimum GP appointments cannot be less than 395.5 million in England.

Realistically, the deficit is 395.5 million minus existing 164 million = 231.5 million appointments.

Let us now find out how many full-time additional GPs, the NHS General Practice in England would need to provide the additional 231.5 million appointments annually.

The maximum number of appointments that one full-time GP can offer per week = 162

(18 appointments per session 9 sessions a week)

Number of appointments one full-time GP can offer over 12 months = 7,452 (162 appointments x 46 weeks; six weeks of holiday)

The big question: How many full-time GPs does the NHS General Practice need to fill the deficit of 231.5 million appointments?

Answer: 231.5 million appointments divided by the number of appointments one full-time GP can offer over the 12 months, which is 7,452

So, 231,500,000/7,452 = 31,065 full time GPs

The figure produced is the result of weeks of research. It is unbelievable that the General Practice in England requires 31,065 more full-time GPs to be able to offer the number of appointments required in one calendar year for the people in England.

Question: If NHS England should continue its policy to have 75 % of its GPs working part-time, how many GPs will the NHS require to recruit?

The shocking answer is: 98,241 Part Time GPs

Calculation:
Number of full time GPs (working 37.5 hours)
= 8,476 (NHS Digital)

Number of all qualified GPs to exclude locums and registrars
= 26,805 (NHS Digital)

Number of additional GPs required as per my calculation
= 31,065

If the NHS continues its policy of 75.7% of its GPs to work part-time, then to have the equivalent of 31,065 full-time GPs the NHS would need: 26,805 divided by 8,476 multiplied by 31,065 = A total GP workforce of 98,241.7

This information is accurate, to the best of my knowledge. Everyone living in England on average sees the GP seven times over a 12-month period. This information comes from the prestigious College of General Practitioners. This figure is pivotal to the total number of GP appointments required. I have double-checked the equally important figure provided by the BMA that of all the GP appointments, only 54.6 % are with the GP Doctors. The remaining 45.4 % are with the non-GP healthcare staff.

For the first time ever, I have been able to pinpoint why the General Practice in England is in a state of nearly irreversible collapse; 230 million additional appointments annually, needing 31,065 full-time GPs are required to have any possibility of people getting prompt medical attention from a GP doctor. If the current tradition of 75 % part-time GP workforce persists, the NHS would need to recruit an additional workforce of 98,241 GPs.

Chapter Eight

My research findings have left me in a state of shock. I have checked my statistics and findings several times and I'm certain that the NHS General Practice is short of 231.5 million GP appointments over 12 months. The consequences of this deficit never discovered by anyone before are devastating.

I had started to write this book to present a credible solution to the misery of millions of people unable to secure a prompt GP appointment, forced to get treatment by telephone from the notorious 111 or head to A&E. I cannot see, what recommendations I can make to fill this unfathomable gap between what the NHS has now and what is realistically required.

What recommendations could I possibly make to recruit 31,065 additional full-time GPs when NHS England has been unable to add even 5,000 GPs over 5 years? Most worrying is that NHS England, academics of the Royal College of General Practitioners, the three NHS related think tanks, with vast human and financial resources have not been able to identify and point out this catastrophe.

It was distressing to note that if the existing policy of 75% part-timers be allowed to run the General Practice in England, then the need to have the required number of GPs would be 98,241. I'm repeating this because I want to share with you my sense of helplessness that's come about through my own research efforts.

I tried to find out the role and numbers of Advance Nurse Practitioners and Physician Associates in the General Practice, to see if they could possibly help.

Advance Nurse Practitioners (ANPs): these are nurses with level 7 MSc qualification in clinical assessment. This includes:

- history taking
- physical examination
- independent prescribing

(Care Quality Commission; ANPs in Primary Care)

It came as a surprise to discover that in several GP practices, the ANPs were seeing and treating people independent of GP supervision and referring them to secondary care where required. Interestingly, the only GP related duty they are not allowed to perform is to issue a sick note or a fit note. Some GP practices that allowed me access to information about the role of ANPs in their practice accepted that the ANPs were undertaking full consultation sessions with no GP supervision.

I asked the question, "could ANPs in the medium to long-term replace the GPs altogether?" This was met with derision. But there did seem to be an acceptance that the ANPs could add significantly to the number of Primary Care appointments. It appears that employing ANPs at half the cost of a 'salaried GP' is one of many strategic tools used to reduce the GP contractors' own workload, thus enabling more off time and increased profitability of the practice. I was amused by the defensive mode of the GPs, who appeared to be concerned about the possibility of their own roles threated and diluted by the ANPs and their status diminished. The NHS England while acknowledging and praising ANPs, who they say, "have shown to improve patient satisfaction and provide high quality care," could only be bothered to add "they alleviate pressures on the GPs".

The NHS has at present 3,931 Advance Nurse Practitioners working in the General Practice. (NHS Digital)

Physician Associates (PAs): on qualification, PAs can see patients in their own appointment slots, formulate a differential diagnosis and develop a patient-centred management plan. They are currently unable to prescribe but are trained in clinical therapeutics and are therefore able to prepare prescriptions for their supervising GPs to sign. (British Journal of General Practice; Role of PAs in general practice)

The Physician Associates can provide medicines by a 'Patient Specific Direction'. It is likely they will gain prescribing privileges in the next few years. (Care Quality Commission; Physician Associates in General Practice)

There are 412 Physician Associates, working in the GP practices (NHS Digital).

Currently, 29 universities are offering training courses and it is estimated there are 1,200 PAs in training.

Unfortunately, the dilemma of 231.5 million GP appointment shortages cannot be met by introducing the ANPs and PAs in the immediate future due to reduced availability, right now.

Gosh! How to introduce in the General Practice in England 31,065 additional full-time GPs or 98,241 additional GPs, if the existing policy of 75% of the workforce were to continue to work part-time!

At this point I felt very sorry for myself, as I had to face the possibility of not finishing this book, unless I was able to find a viable solution. I was in a stalemate situation.

- Operated by the GPs, 75 % of whom work part time only (NHS Digital)
- Denying face-to-face consultations to their registered patients after 6 pm Monday to Friday, Saturdays, and Sundays.
- Forcing them to receive treatment by telephone through the notorious NHS 111, 118 hours every week of the year
- Making people wait two weeks for an appointment (National average, survey, Pulse)
- Short of 31,065 full time GPs (Chapter Eight)
- The only public service in the world which though totally funded by the taxpayers, is run for profit by GP contractors and private companies

The NHS General Practice in England is a
'FAILED ESSENTIAL PUBLIC SERVICE'

SOLUTION?

The General Practice Revolution

Chapter Nine

The Dawn of Revolutiq; from the 'season of darkness to the season of light, from the winter of despair to the spring of hope'. A light at the end of the tunnel.

The novelists call it writers' block, the inability to continue with writing as everything seems to have come to a dead end. In my case, it felt like a 'full stop'. One cannot use imagination and play on words in a scientific treatise. I was unable to present a solution based on my own research that the General Practice in England requires an additional 31,065 GPs at best and 98,241 at worst to be able to offer the required appointments. From where are these doctors going to come from and how?

For an agonising five months, I did not and frankly could not write a single sentence. And then out of the blue I stumbled across some facts, which made me cry out, 'Eureka!'

This is what I found out.

1. 40% of all the GP appointments are related to mental health issues (mind.org.uk)
2. 30 % of GP appointments are for musculoskeletal conditions (NHS England)

Mental Health Issues:

- People with mental health issues constitute 40% of all the GP appointments.
- GPs do not have the expertise to deal with them. Every GP I talked to agrees with this!

- The average length of an appointment (10 minutes) makes the job frustrating to the GP and next to useless to the sufferer.

NHS England has already started a Pilot Programme 'IAPT', Improving Access to Psychological Therapy, employing Psychological Wellbeing Practitioners (PWP). Starting in 2008, the IAPT programme is now seeing 900,000 people a year and is committed to further expanding to 1.5 million people. The impressive list of mental health problems covered include:

Depression, generalised anxiety disorder, social anxiety disorder, panic disorder, agoraphobia, obsessive-compulsive disorder, specific phobias, PTSD, hypochondriasis etc.

The Improving Access to Psychological Therapies Manual has been produced by the National Collaborating Centre for Mental Health, on behalf of NHS England, (first published in June 2018 and updated March 2020). The outcomes are documented and impressive:

'Currently approximately one in two people who have a course of treatment in IAPT recover and two out of three people show worthwhile improvements in their mental health.' (NHS England)

GPs do not have the training or expertise to deal with mental health problems of this complexity, except to hand over a prescription for tranquilisers or anti-depressants. The outcomes are devastating to those suffering from such a wide range of mental health problems. In today's era of super specialisation, to expect a GP to offer treatment to those with mental health problems, is like asking a skin specialist to undertake brain surgery!

Musculoskeletal Problems in the General Practice.
My research confirmed that:

- 30% of all the GP consultations are related to back pain, neck pain, bone pain, muscle pain and joint pain.
- Unfortunately, for the sufferers the only treatment a GP can offer is pain killers, which is like using a sticking plaster to cure a fracture.
- Physiotherapy can help to manage, reduce, and significantly improve the symptoms of those in chronic pain with arthritis and similar Musculoskeletal Problems.

NHS England has started a pilot scheme in 41 areas providing 'physiotherapists with enhanced skills' called 'Musculoskeletal Practitioners' (MSK). These are patients 'first and direct contact, without involving GPs'. Findings from 6,800 MSK appointments showed good outcomes. Those treated were:

- less likely to have blood tests or drug prescriptions
- less likely to be referred to consultant-led services with 21% fewer referrals to hospital orthopaedic services.
- 99% gave positive feedback.

The Musculoskeletal Practitioners are qualified autonomous clinical practitioners, who are able to assess, diagnose, treat, and discharge a person without a GP appointment.
(NHS England)

Analyses of 2 years data of 8,417 patients' outcomes concluded:
"The patients with musculoskeletal conditions may be assessed and managed independently and effectively by the

Musculoskeletal Practitioners instead of GPs."
(pubmed.ncbi.nlm.nih.gov)

The Bombshell Recommendation to change the General Practice in England for ever:

Allow 40 % of the appointments to be treated by the Psychological-wellbeing Practitioners (PWP), 30 % by the Musculoskeletal Practitioners (MSK) and let the GPs treat the remaining 30% of total appointments.

These can be further reduced by using the current NHS Advance Nurse Practitioners and Physician Associates (Chapter Eight).

At first glance this may look strange. And yet, specialisation and super specialisation has transformed the modern secondary health care in hospitals. The field of medicine no longer has one dedicated physician, surgery no longer one dedicated surgeon. Let me give you an example. In the good old days, Orthopaedic Surgery was one speciality to deal with all surgical problems relating to "bones and joints". Now the super specialisation has one dedicated surgeon for the cervical spine, one for the lumbar and thoracic spine, one for hips only, one for shoulders only, one for hands only, one for the ankles only. The running joke amongst the orthopaedic surgeons is "soon I would be dealing only with the right knee and my colleague with the left knee". I brought to your attention earlier that there are over sixty specialties practiced by the super specialists in hospitals.

Unfortunately, no such division has occurred in the NHS General Practice. My in-depth research indicates conclusively that the GPs are ill-trained to treat complex mental health problems and musculoskeletal conditions. I have interviewed several GPs and everyone without exception has accepted that the non-GP Healthcare professionals could be the best to offer the initial treatment and involve them only if necessary.

So, this changes dramatically the main problem of the shortage of GPs.

If the GPs are dealing with 30% of all appointments only, how many full-time GPs does the NHS General Practice in England require?

Calculation:
Considering that on average one person consults a GP seven times in 12 months, the total number of GP appointments required, for the population in England of 56.5 million people:

56.5 million x 7 = 395,500,000 appointments over 12 months.

Of these, the proposed appointments with the GP doctors would be 30 %,

395,500,000 x 30% = 118,650,000

At the time of writing there are 3,931 Advance Nurse Practitioners (ANPs) working in the GP practices in England. If everyone were to be asked to work full-time, producing ten sessions a week, an additional 180 appointments a week can be generated per ANP per week.

Let us be on the cautious side and consider on average each ANP produces only 150 appointments instead of 180.

Calculation:
150 appointments a week x 46 working weeks = 6,900

So, number of new appointments created from 3,931 ANPs 6,900 x 3,931 = 27,123,900

30% of all appointments with GPs as established
= 118,650,000

Number of appointments which the ANPs can share with GPs
= 27,123,900

Number of appointments which only GPs would do
= 118,650,000 minus 27,123,900

= 91,526,100 appointments

The number of appointments that one full time GP offers per week = 162 (18 appointments per session 9 sessions a week)

Number of appointments one full time GP can offer over 12 months = 7,452 (162 appointments x 46 weeks; 6weeks holidays)

Number of Full Time GPs required to offer 91,526,100 appointments over 12 months

91,526,100 divided by 7,452 = 12,282.08 Full Time GPs.

The Eureka Moment:

If GPs offered consultations to just 30% of all appointments, which they are best able to cope with, the NHS General Practice would require only 12,282 full-time GPs, helped by the existing 3,931 Advance Nurse Practitioners (ANPs)

(31,065 full-time or 98,241 part-time additional GPs required, Chapter Seven).

Considering that the total number of all GPs to include locums and registrars is 35,273 (NHS Digital), the General Practice in England could have a surplus of 22,991 GPs.
35,273 minus 12,282 = 22,991

This surplus of GPs should be more than capable of providing the treatment to people of England after 6pm, and on weekends, through a structured reallocation of the resources. No one can deny that this arrangement would produce dramatically better outcomes through early diagnosis and treatment, saving lives.

Let us now find out how many Psychological Wellbeing Practitioners (PWP) are required to take over 40 % of the GP appointments. I have recommended 20 minutes for each appointment and 21 appointments a day; Mon- Fri.
The NHS England would require 32,753 total Psychological Wellbeing Practitioners (PWP)

Calculation:
395,500,000 annual GP appointments required x 40%
= 158,200,000 appointments

20 minutes appointment for each person and 21 appointments in a day, 11 in the morning and 10 in the afternoon sessions

21 appointments x 20 minutes = 420 minutes = 7 hours and spare 30 minutes if one appointment spills over.

21 appts a day x 5 days a week = 105 a week

105 a week x 46 weeks = 4,830 over 12 months (6 weeks holidays)

158,200,000 / 4,830 = 32,753.62 PWPs needed

Let us now find out how many Musculoskeletal Practitioners are required to take over 30 % of the GP appointments. I have recommended 20 minutes for each appointment and 21 appointments a day, Mon- Fri.

Calculation:
I hope you remember that the NHS General Practice needs 395 million appointments by the people of England.

395,500,000 x 30% = 1118,650,000 appointments (to be dealt with by the Musculoskeletal Practitioners).

20-minute appointments for each person and 21 appointments a day, 11 in the morning and 10 in the afternoon sessions

21 appointments x 20 minutes = 420 minutes = 7 hours and spare 30 minutes if one appointment spills over.

21 appts a day x 5 a week = 105

105 a week x 46 = 4,830 (6 weeks holidays) over 12 months .

118,650,000 / 4,830 = 24,565.21

24,565 Musculoskeletal Practitioners (MSK) needed.

It is the ultimate reward of my efforts and research to discover that the NHS England, has no GP shortage and requires only 12,282 full-time GPs, if 40% of all the Mental Health matters of the General Practice in England are dealt with by the Psychological Welfare Practitioners and 30% of the Musculoskeletal Problems by the MSK Practitioners, as the Direct Access Professionals, helped by 3,931 APNs already working in GP practices in England.

For the first time in the seventy years history of the Primary Care in England, I have demonstrated how the entire structure of the General Practice can be 'turned around' by transferring 70% of the GPs responsibilities to Direct Access Professionals. This would allow the GPs to do what they are trained to best deal with and put an end to their historical shortages. More importantly, people with mental health problems and musculoskeletal problems will have prompt, 'no wait' attention with superior outcomes.

It is worth noting that if the number of ANPs is increased from 3,139 to just 5,000, the number of GPs needed is further reduced to 11,292.

Oh, what if the number of ANP's is increased to 8,000? Remember, in every GP practice, the ANPs are seeing patients face-to-face, making a diagnosis, issuing prescriptions, referring to hospital consultants without GP supervision. The Physician Associates with existing small numbers but significantly more in the training process are already playing a valuable role in the General Practice.

Bring in more ANPs, add Physician Associates and the historical and desperate shortage of GPs will turn into a surplus. The scarcity of GPs will disappear forever. The combined force of GPs, Direct Access Professionals, ANP's, Physician Associates would provide, same day, face-to-face consultations, 8 am to 6 pm, after 6 pm and the weekends, 24/7.

Is this a miracle?

No, it is the NHS General Practice Revolution.

Chapter Ten

Seven Steps of the General Practice Revolution.

New dawn will come and then the unvanquished humanity will trace the path of conquest, despite all barriers"
(Nobel prize winner R.N. Tagore)

I had telephone conversations with many people including, the NHS hospital consultants, GPs, nurses, acquaintances, friends, and my own family. I also spoke to readers of my book 'NHS is Not Working' who had kindly communicated with me. I wanted to have their views if the NHS England General Practice could be radically reformed by providing a credible and workable solution, with the following goal:

"The General Practice in England should provide prompt face-to-face GP consultations to people during the day and same day availability for semi-urgent problems arising after 6pm and over the weekend."

Here is a sample of three responses, representing most of them:

"What greater service can anyone do to all of us in England than what you are proposing to! Go ahead. I fully support you. It won't be easy."

"It is time, someone helps my family and millions like us to be able to get a prompt face-to-face GP appointment. If you have a young child needing medical attention, then the only way to avoid the hideous treatment by telephone from the NHS 111 is to sit for 6 hours in the A&E to see a doctor. Please go ahead. I wish you the best."

"If you can present a genuine solution to this horrible problem, affecting every one of us, it would be a revolution, for which, I believe the time has now come. You have my blessings and backing."

This chapter is about radical reform of the NHS General Practice. I would describe a complete framework of how this can be accomplished in a logical, scientific, evidence-based list of steps. No guesswork, no wishful thinking. Rene Descartes, the French philosopher, mathematician, and scientist famously said, "we must further realise that while the discovery of an 'order' is no easy task, once the order has been discovered, there is no difficulty at all in knowing it."

Rene Descartes ('I think; therefore, I am') was the inventor of analytical geometry, linking the previous separate fields of geometry and algebra.

Like the whodunnit detective story, I would use all the clues from the previous chapters in a logical "step by step" methodology.

I revealed that unlike a hospital, delivering highly advanced sets of treatments through sophisticated equipment and operating theatres costing millions of pounds, a GP's old-fashioned surgery premises or awe-inspiring health centre is just a brick-and-mortar building, like any office, with the small possibility of a two-year-old ECG machine as its most expensive and sophisticated piece of equipment. And truthfully, all a GP requires to offer a 10-minute consultation is an eight-by-eight feet office with a hand wash basin, a stethoscope, a BP measuring instrument, a desk, a computer, gloves, an examination couch, chairs for patients and nothing more. (Chapter Three)

I have put an end to the great lie that the General Practice is a highly complex structure, which can only be effectively managed by the 'profit hungry' private companies or the GP contractors, and only if they can make huge profits from the taxpayers.

I have exposed the breath-taking incompetence of the NHS England in not knowing how many more GPs are required to fulfil the basic obligations of the GPs to their registered patients. I have revealed that whereas everyone agrees on GP shortages as a major problem, no one knows the accurate number required. Figures of 4,000, 5,000, 6,000, 9,000 are thrown in the air. Worst, no one seems to know what goal would be achieved by more GPs. These are all observations, comments, opinions with no evidence to support, confirming what Bertrand Russell famously pointed out, "The fact that an opinion has been widely held, is no evidence whatever that it is not but utterly absurd."

All I communicate to you is based on evidence. No wild hypotheses, no imaginative theories.

I pointed out that to determine the exact number of GPs required, one must calculate the number of appointments needed by the 56.5 million people of England. I was the first ever to discover after extensive research that the number of additional full-time GPs required, if no changes are made would be, 31,065. I disclosed to you that 75% GPs work part-time in sharp contrast to only 25% of the employees working part-time in the UK and horror of horrors, a massive 98,241 more GPs would be required if the current policy of part-time GPs employment is to be maintained. (Chapter Seven)

Finally, I demonstrated that if 70% of all GP appointments are dealt with by the Direct Access Professionals, helped by 3,193

Advance Nurse Practitioners, the NHS General Practice needs only 12,282 full-time GPs. Increase the number of ANPs from the existing 3,193 to just 5,000, and the number of total full-time GPs required falls to 11,292.

SEVEN STEPS TO THE
NHS GENERAL PRACTICE REVOLUTION:

Step One -
Abolish the self-employed status of GPs. Give them a fair salary like their hospital colleagues. The NHS should take back control of the General Practice, which is currently owned, managed and run for profit by GP contractors and private companies. This step alone would allow the taxpayers funded General Practice to save millions of pounds made as profit by the private companies and the GP contractors.

I repeat my challenge to anyone to show me one public sector in England, which is a source of multimillion pound profits by the private companies and where the employees can make 3-4 times more than the UK Prime Minister, all at the expense of the taxpayer. The complex structure of payments to a GP practice based on the number of people registered with it would be abolished.

The extraordinary manoeuvres by the NHS management to pay remuneration to the GP Practices, so that the GP contractors and private companies can make huge profits by using salaried doctors, locums, advance nurse practitioners and a mushrooming number of staff would be reviewed and eliminated.

It would be the responsibility of NHS England to employ new GPs in areas where they are needed and not the private companies or the GP contractors. No longer will deprived

areas have a situation where their General Practices are being closed, because they're no longer in the commercial interests of the 'profit mongers'.
(54 GPs per 100,000 people, Northwest London; 69 GPs per 100,000 people Southwest Chapter One.)

An equitable and generous new contract of employment would be offered to 25 % of the GPs who work full-time and 75% to those who work 'part-time'. The salaries would be calculated on the number of sessions that a GP offers, and the agreed number of people offered face-to-face consultations in each session and NOT, based on the number of people who had the misfortune to be handcuffed to the GP Practices through registration with a GP contractor. (Chapter Five)

This would create greater job satisfaction for most GPs. They would be employed and paid by the NHS and not by the GP contract-masters or the private companies managed and owned by the layman investors.

Evidence suggests new, young doctors are put off and demoralised by the demands to manage finances and business as they are not trained for it. Becoming a GP contractor seems to be the only way to avoid employment on depressed wages as a salaried-GP. By making them NHS salaried, bringing them in line with hospital doctors, this problem would no longer exist.

Step Two -
Give choice to all the GPs "Work for the NHS General Practice or for the Private Companies, not both!

The 25 % full-time GPs would be reminded that they cannot be allowed to work additional hours for the private companies when they claim to be too overworked and stressed to offer appointments to their own registered patients for two weeks.

The 75% part-time GPs must spend all their available time to their NHS patients and not use the NHS as a platform to generate money by working for the private companies whilst enjoying all the benefits of NHS employment. They would be welcome to offer more sessions to see more NHS patients and generate more money if this is the reason for their part-time choice. GPs retain their rights to resign from the NHS and work for the private companies.

Here's a very important point that merits repeating:

"Every GP helping to generate multi-million pounds profit for the private companies, is fully employed by the NHS on a generous salary, has gold-plated pension, six weeks of holiday and sick pay benefits"

Well-known horror stories where people who were unable to get an appointment for two weeks from their own practice, were able to secure a next day private appointment from the very same practice doctor or a partner, through a private company, are ethically and morally repugnant, loathsome, and unacceptable.

Before I proceed with the Step Three, let me please tell you the tale of a builder, given a contract to build a house in Wales by a rich Londoner. After three years, the house was still not built. The report commissioned by the owner from a Building Consultant for this unacceptable delay was as follows:

The builder is hard working and honest and is suffering from stress caused by the delay. Unfortunately, he is doing all the work himself.

He is laying bricks; he is not a trained bricklayer though very knowledgeable on the subject.

He is plastering walls; he is not a plasterer, though very knowledgeable on the subject.

He is installing plumbing; he is not a plumber, though very knowledgeable on the subject.

He is doing all the electrics; he is not an electrician, though very knowledgeable on the subject.

He has been constructing the roof; he is not a roofer, though very knowledgeable on the subject.

We recommend, appropriate tradesmen; plasterers, plumbers, electricians, roofers to do the specialised tasks. (Signed Jeremy Boden, Boden & Co Building Consultants)

The NHS GP is that builder. He has no expertise in mental health problems constituting 40% of all his appointments but sees the people with these anyway, dishing them tons of tranquilisers and antidepressants. He has no expertise in musculoskeletal problems constituting 30% of all his appointments but sees the people with these anyway, prescribing tons of pain killers and NSAIDs (Non-Steroid Anti-Inflammatory Drugs)

Step Three -
Seventy per cent of all the NHS GP appointments would be handled by 'Direct Access Professionals'.

People needing medical advice and treatment will be able to make appointments directly with the relevant professionals, without contacting GPs first:

- All mental health matters with Psychological Welfare Professionals and not the GPs (Constituting 40% of all GP appointments)
- All bone, joint, muscle pain problems with the Musculoskeletal Professionals and not the GPs. (Constituting 30% of all GP appointments)
- Rest of the health problems with the Doctor General Practitioners, Advance Nurse Practitioners, Physician Associates. (Constituting 30% of all GP appointments)

No one would ever consider requesting a hip replacement from a respiratory physician nor expect treatment of an eye condition from a skin specialist. Why, should it be expected from a GP to treat people with mental health and musculoskeletal problems, with none or very limited expertise? It would come as a huge relief to the GPs to transfer the burden of 70% of all appointments to those with the specialised knowledge and skills.

This step is a genuine revolution in the way the General Practice in England is provided. It opens floodgates to a variety of primary healthcare services, through 'Direct Access Professionals', without a GP consultation.

All eye problems can be, and frankly should be, dealt with by 'Direct Access Optometrist Professionals'. I can confirm that no GP, to my knowledge, has a slit lamp device to diagnose eye conditions, nor any training to use it. The optometrists would be a part of the Appointments Portals, as described in chapter four. They could continue to practise from their own premises but offer the NHS appointments for the symptoms related to eye conditions but not for routine eye tests for glasses.

Female patients can make appointments with the Direct Access female nurse professionals to have initial consultation for gynaecological and breast problems. Males should be able to make appointments with Direct Access male Physician Associates professional for a routine medical health check, to include prostate and any other personal problems, which they may feel shy about.

The goal here is to make the non-GP professionals in the General Practice available to the people with medical concerns easily and promptly and without consultation with the GPs. The role of the GPs remains undiminished. They would continue to diagnose, investigate, treat, and refer.

I described in chapter nine that NHS England, has no GP shortage and requires only 12,282 full-time GPs, if 40% of all the Mental Health matters of the General Practice in England are dealt with by the Psychological Welfare Practitioners and 30% of the Musculoskeletal Problems by the MSK Practitioners, as the Direct Access Professionals, helped by 3,931 APNs already working in GP practices in England.

Suddenly, the unfathomable deficit of GPs disappears. The market forces with demand outstripping the supply is blown to smithereens. The oft repeated excuses by the NHS Management, explanations by the academics and the think tanks, declaring GP shortages as the main reason for the dreadful Primary Care being provided to the people of England, suddenly withers away. I will explain later how the surplus of GPs thus created could be utilised.

One of the most important steps of the 'GP Revolution' is to open the General Practice to everyone, so that they can seek quick medical attention, denied to millions of people unable to secure a prompt GP appointment. This has already put a barrier to most people seeking help, leading to late diagnosis and considerably worse outcomes.

- 22% out of 365,000 people found to have cancer, were diagnosed in A&E (Cancer Research UK)
- 40 % of people with lung cancer first reached specialist care through A&E (UK Lung Cancer Coalition)

A consultant oncologist commented:
" These outrageous findings are a matter of disgrace, for the General Practice in England, and living proof that people are meeting an early and avoidable death because they are unable to get a GP appointment. People's only way to get face-to-face medical attention now appears to be through Accident & Emergency departments."

Step Four -
Abolish with urgency the NHS 111. Chapter Five has been devoted to the service which provides treatment by telephone, 110 hours a week out of 168, employing non-medically qualified people with 6 weeks training. By its 24/7 availability, NHS England has openly acknowledged and confessed that the GPs in England are no longer available to provide appointments to their registered patients even Mondays to Fridays, 8am to 6pm.

The existence and operations of the NHS 111 is an abomination and a slur on Primary Care. It must be dismantled and be replaced by face-to-face consultations with a professional. I will explain in detail, how this can be achieved, both operationally and financially.

Step Five -
Replace phone requests for an appointment with an online

appointment system. I have explained in detail in Chapter Four the introduction of the Monday to Friday online appointments portal system to replace the existing antiquated telephone method and the introduction of an out of hours and weekend online appointments portal system.

Of course, facilities would be made available to help a small minority of the people unable to make online appointments. The only change from then is the addition of online portals to include the ability to make direct appointments with the:

- Direct Access Psychological Welfare professionals
- Direct Access Musculoskeletal professionals
- Direct Access Optometrists professionals
- Direct Access female nurse professionals
- Direct Access GP professionals
- Direct Access Advance Nurse professionals
- Direct Access Physician Associates professionals.

Through this step, for the first time in the history of General Practice in England, Primary Care would offer abundant, easy and prompt appointments. The current rationing and scarcity, to deter the fearful people with health anxieties to seek medical attention would turn to a reassuring and welcoming service provided by an array of non-GP professionals and GPs themselves.

Step Six -
Regulate the private sector that provides the General Practice Services. Funded 100% by the Government, the NHS General Practice is a nationalised public service, where the profit motive should never be the primary objective. Miraculously it

embraces both the Keynesian and the laissez- faire economic models but amazingly and disastrously, has no accountability to the end users or the funders. And worse, no fear of failure or bankruptcy on account of incompetence.

I have discussed at length the involvement of private companies in Chapter Two. There are two types of private companies offering their services. The first kind promises a same day or next-day appointment by phone, video or face-to-face on payment to a GP.

The other has been allowed to enter the infrastructure of the General Practice through NHS reforms. You may have read in the press how one private individual has applied for a judicial review into awarding of dozens of NHS GP contracts to Operose, a subsidiary of a US company, Centene, which has acquired 52 GP practices across England. I have been unable to find out how NHS England has allowed the entirely taxpayer-funded General Practice to be taken over by private companies. This obviously has been made possible by allowing the GP contractors to have a sham self-employed status, allowing them to buy or sell their practices. Terminating this self-employed status and making every GP a salaried doctor should put an end to this.

There is no evidence to show that the international companies based in tax havens and the US, making millions of pounds of profit for their shareholders, employing taxpayer-funded (moon lighting) NHS GPs, using NHS-paid practice staff, housed in NHS rent-paid practice premises, are providing a better standard of medical care to the people, than the vast majority of the rest of the practices in England run by the GP contractors.

I have shown repeatedly that the General Practice operations are simple and do not need management by the private companies, funded by the national and international investors. I would recommend no bar or restriction to the operations of private companies wanting to offer any kind of the service relating to General Practice except fair and equitable regulations:

1. No private company may employ a GP or a doctor working in the NHS part-time or full-time. The doctors must be on full payroll of the private company.
2. The doctors offering private GP services to the private companies must have a clearance from the NHS on their professional capability and a regular review of their competence to keep up with the latest academic developments.
3. The private GPs cannot write the NHS prescriptions, and their patients must pay for the prescribed medicines at the going market rate. In addition, all investigations to include blood tests, X-rays, scans etc., must be paid and cannot be offered on free NHS.

Chapter Eleven

Step - Seven

The NHS General Practice Revolution will deliver "Prompt, 'No Wait', Face-to-Face GP Consultations to people during the day and same-day availability for semi-urgent and urgent problems arising after 6pm and over the weekend". An end to the nonsense that for 110 hours of 168 in a week, people in England should receive treatment by telephone only from a call centre.

The NHS General Practice Revolution would get rid of all the barriers to receiving medical attention. The unfortunate philosophy of the NHS management now engraved in their DNA is that people need to contact their GP only if essential and must wait for two weeks. This would be eliminated.

It is now well-established that hindrances to getting an early GP appointment leads to late diagnosis and notably worse outcomes. My research indicates that a significant number of people are deterred from seeking medical attention by the disingenuous PR and policies by the NHS with the slogan, 'Why do you want to see the GP?'. While feeling guilty, if the people 'dare' to 'abuse' their General Practice's allegedly overloaded system, they find it difficult to get an early GP appointment.

"66% of adults have chosen to delay or put off making an appointment, resulting in catastrophic consequences. 41% admitted they feel negative about going to the doctors. 29% said going to see their GP makes them anxious and nervous." (Research conducted by YouGov on behalf of Co-Op Health)

You may remember that in Chapter Nine, I explained that by minimising the number of GP consultations to just 30%, we have an astonishing scenario of 22,991 surplus GPs.

Let us calculate how many new appointments would be created from the 'newfound' workforce of 22,991 GPs. My research shows that no part-time GP works fewer than two days a week, offering four consultation sessions and 72 appointments a week. With six weeks holiday, 46 weeks over 12 months.

Calculation:
72 appointments a week over 46 weeks:
46 x 72 = 3,312 appointments over 12 months per GP

Number of new appointments created from 22,991 GPs:
3,312 x 22,991 = 76,146,192

At the time of writing there are 3,931 Advance Nurse Practitioners (ANPs) working in the GP practices in England. If everyone were to be asked to work full-time, producing ten sessions a week, an additional 180 appointments a week can be generated per ANP per week.

Let us be on the cautious side and consider on average each ANP produces only 150 appointments instead of 180

Calculation:
150 appointments a week x 46 working weeks = 6,900

Number of new appointments created from 3,931 ANPs:
6,900 x 3,931 = 27,123,900

Grand Total of new additional appointments:
76,146,192 + 27,123,900 = 103,270,092

Let us now calculate how many appointments the NHS 111 offers, 24/7 for every medical problem of the General Practice in England, which the GPs in England do not deal with:

Calculation:
The NHS 111 offers on average 57,000 appointments to people a day (NHS England).

The total number of appointments over 365 days:
57,000 x 365 = 20,805,500 (over 12 months)

Number of new appointments generated as per above calculation: 103,270,092 over 12 months.

Number of appoints offered by the NHS 111
= 20,805,500 over 12 months.

By dismantling the NHS 111, we have 82,464,592 surplus appointments (103,270,092 minus 20,805,500 = 82,464,592)

These 82,464,592 face-to-face' appointments, after the abolition of NHS 111 can offer:

- Daytime Monday to Friday no-wait appointments
- Semi-urgent and urgent medical problems arising after 6pm, on Saturdays and Sundays through the online appointments portal system (Chapter Four)

The fundamental change involved in the General Practice Revolution is to bring back the work ethic of the doctors in General Practice in line with those of their hospital colleagues, available 24 hours a day, 7 days a week.

Every hospital doctor, whether house officer, senior house officer, registrar, senior registrar, or a consultant must do a certain number of 'after hours' work to include night duties and weekends over the 12-month period. I am recommending a similar though less strenuous workload for every General Practitioner, working full-time or part-time. Here is a report of hospital doctors on duty 'after hours' from two reliable resources, stipulating that 'there is no national standard format for it and different hospitals may have different pattern.' I copy the information as provided:

Source one: consultant surgeon on call does 36 nights in a year and six weekends starting from Friday morning finishing on Monday afternoon.

Source two: rota for Senior Fellows and Registrars:

20 long weekdays:	7.45 to 19.45; 12 hours
20 weekday nights:	7.30pm to 8 am; 12 hours 30 minutes
15 weekend nights:	7.30 to 8 am; 12 hours 30 minutes
15 weekend days:	7.45 am to 19.45 pm; 12 hours

The restoration of working after 6pm and on weekends is only possible by abolishing the pseudo status of GP self-employment. As employees of the NHS the GPs must comply to the working practices of doctors prevalent in all hospitals in England. The employees of the Essential Public Services have no such nonsense as 'opting out' and working office hours.

In my book 'NHS is not Working' one of my main recommendations is to decentralise the operations of the NHS to small regional units, each supervised with the help of the local captains of industry and local people. This guiding principle remains one of the foundation's pillars. We know that each city, town and village has its local GP practices and the vast majority of the population has access to a GP practice within 10 to 15 miles.

The NHS management with new powers, would arrange a certain number of GP practices to pool their patients geographically, covering a population number of say 30,000 – 50,000 people, offering a service through the out of hours and weekend online appointments portals from nominated surgery or health centre premises. A region with this kind of a population of 300,000 to 500,000 could be served by 10 centres or more.

The shifts for the GPs, in each of the health centres/ surgery premises would be:

- 6pm to 9 pm
- 9pm to 12 midnight
- 12 midnight to 8 am

The appointments would be through the online portals (Chapter Four) and telephone facilities available strictly to those with no internet access. No GP will do more than six weekends (four sessions of three hours), six sessions 6pm-9pm, six sessions 9pm-12 midnight and only two-night duties in a 12-month period.

I am confident that by careful planning of the additional appointments made available, the NHS General Practice would be restored to an Essential 24/7 Primary Care Service, providing prompt appointments during the weekdays and same-day appointments for semi-urgent and urgent problems arising after 6pm and weekends, similar to other essential public services like fire, ambulance, hospitals, police.

An amusing cartoon appeared in a newspaper. The shoppers on arrival at a supermarket serving 24/7 to their customers note a big sign stating:

SORRY
We do not serve GPs after 6pm
and not at all on
Saturdays and Sundays

Chapter Twelve

The principal excuse for the failings of the General Practice is claimed to be a shortage of money; NHS England has never provided an accurate figure, nor what goals and objectives would be achieved as a solution if the required funds were provided.

Instead, the concepts and policies dreamt by NHS England to centralise the GP Practices to 1,250 large Primary Care Networks (PCN's) are brandished. The abstract ramblings of the NHS England, not for the benefit of the long-suffering people of England but rather a narcissistic non, evidence-based habit to confuse the public, are being presented as an answer. The new buzz word of 'integrated care systems', provides a great opportunity to bamboozle.

Here seems to be the solution to the General Practice problems:

"The Primary Care Networks (PCN's) will be required to deliver a set of seven national service specifications...they are 'building blocks of Integrated Care Systems (ICS). The first consideration is how the voice of PCNs can most effectively be brought into ICS or Sustainability and Transformation Plans (STPs) in other areas" (Abstract article Anna Charles, King's Fund.)

Absolutely nowhere in this self-congratulatory plethora of vague verbosity can there be found any mention of how the people in England could be helped to access 'no wait' 24/7 GP consultations.

I would address the fundamental questions, never raised, or answered in the last 30 years. What is the projected funding deficit of the NHS General Practice? What goals and objectives would be achieved if this funding deficit is met? Can all or some of the required funds be raised?

Based on a 20-minute appointment and 21 appointments a day over five days, I have calculated that 32,753 Psychological Wellbeing Practitioners are required to delegate the 40% of all GP appointments relating to mental health problems, and 24,565 Musculoskeletal Practitioners to delegate the 30% of appointments relating to symptoms of pains and aches in muscles, bones, and joints. (Chapter Nine)

Unfortunately, I have not been able to find out how many Psychological Wellbeing Practitioners (PWPs) and Musculoskeletal Practitioners (MSKs) are currently available and practicing in the NHS. The available information gives an idea:

The NHS England has already started a Pilot Programme 'IAPT; Improving Access to Psychological Therapy employing Psychological Wellbeing Practitioners (PWP). Starting in 2008, the IAPT programme is now seeing 900,000 people a year and is committed to further expanding to 1.5 million people.

NHS England has started a pilot scheme in 41 areas providing 'physiotherapists with enhanced skills' called 'Musculoskeletal Practitioners' (MSK). These are patients' first and direct contact, without involving GPs. Findings from 6,800 MSK appointments showed good outcomes.

I have decided to use the cost of employing these professionals as if the NHS had none. Here are my calculations:

Salary structure and cost to the NHS of employing 32,753 Psychological Wellbeing Practitioners (PWPs):
Average salary of a PWP as quoted by several sources:

- £21,692 to £34,876. (opencollnet.org.uk)
- £29,828 (reed.co.uk)
- £25,026 (glassdoor.co.uk)
- £24,157 starting to £30,615 (Band five, prospects.ac.uk)
- Let us calculate on an average of £28,000 annually

Salaries projected cost; 32,753 x 28,000 = £ 917,084,000

Salary structure and cost to the NHS of employing new 24,565 Musculoskeletal Practitioners (MSK):

Average salary of an MSK as quoted by some sources:

- Band seven £38,890 – 44,503 (mft.nhs.uk)
- £38,890 – 44,503 (jobs.wuth.nhs.uk)
- Let us calculate on an average of say £40,00 annually

Salaries projected cost: 24,565 x 40,000 = £982,600,000

Direct Access Psychological Welfare Professionals annual
salaries   = £917,084,000
Direct Access Musculoskeletal Professionals annual
salaries   = £982,600,000

Total   = £ 1,899,684,000
In short, it is roughly £1.9 billion.

I consider it my number one priority to be totally honest and transparent in all that I write in this book. There is a possibility that the amount required to pay the annual salaries of the Direct Access Psychological Welfare Professionals and the Musculoskeletal Professionals may be significantly more if my proposed 20 - minute appointment should be increased to 30 or 40 minutes and adding the national insurance contributions etc.

Let me start with the amount of £1.9 billion required. How can this amount be raised? A macabre witticism; through the death of the NHS 111 and 'exorcism of the ghosts'!

Savings through demise of the NHS 111: request under the Freedom of Information Act from NHS England, NHS Digital and Office of National Statistics states:
'accurate operational cost of running the NHS 111 over 12 months is NOT available.'

Speculating on the turnover figures, I estimate that the cost of operating each NHS 111 centre to be approximately £20 million, based on the following information:

Vocare: three centres; latest accounts turnover, £60,227,874. Nedvivo group: one centre; latest accounts turnover £21,844,629

It appears that the total number of NHS 111 centres in England is 68.
Projected running cost of all NHS 111 centres:
£20 million x 68 = £1,360,000,000. (1billion, 360million)

This figure is based on available facts and appears to be a correct assumption.

Savings through exorcism of ghosts: exorcism (from Greek exorkismos) is the practice of evicting ghosts, from the possessed. I appear to have become a practitioner in the occult. Watch the process of exorcism.

Population of England = 56,500,000
(Office of National Statistics)

Number of people registered with all GP practices in England is 60,970,002 (NHS Digital)

The difference must be ghosts!

Number of 'ghosts' for which GP Practices receive an annual income per person but who do not exist = 4,470,002.

"GP practices were paid on average of £155 per patient in 2019/20" (Pulse magazine)

Annual income of the GP Practices for ghost people on their lists, who do not exist:

4,470,002 x £155 = £692,850,310.

When the GP Practices are no longer paid by the number of people registered with them but by fixed salaries (Chapter Three), the massive sum of £692,850,310 would be saved.

(Please note that except for the NHS, I do not take cases of exorcism, contact your local spiritualist!)

I'm concerned you may think the above information is "fake news". Is it possible for this vast amount of money being paid to the GP practices to look after people who do not exist? The resounding answer is, YES. Both the figures related to the number of all people registered with the GP practices in England from the NHS Digital and the population of England from the ONS are correct.

So amount saved:
From abolition of the NHS 111 = £1,360,000,000

From cessation of payments based on people who do not exist = £692,850,310

Total = £2,052,850,310 annually.
This is in excess of £2 billion.

Total amount of salaries of new Direct Access Psychological Welfare Professionals and Direct Access Musculoskeletal Professionals salaries required is £1,892,412,000, annually

Amount saved:
£2,052,850,310 minus £1,892,412,000 = £160,438,310

This is a saving of over £160.4 million.

Please note that these projections are based on the available facts and consider two factors:

1. Contrary to the information from the NHS England, I have assumed that the NHS does not have even one Psychological Welfare Professional and no Musculoskeletal Professionals.
2. I have stipulated a twenty-minute standard appointment for each consultation. There is a possibility of a longer appointment, thus increasing the number of these two professionals in my projected figures.
3. I have calculated the cost of operating the NHS 111 to be £1,360,000,000.

There is a distinct possibility that currently the number of projected required Psychological Welfare Professionals and Musculoskeletal Professionals may not be available, in the short term. My research indicates that there is a significant number of both the Psychological Welfare Professionals and Musculoskeletal Professionals working in the NHS.

There are enough places in the universities for a desired number to be achieved within a reasonably short period. The Government will have to start a campaign to incentivise the lucrative and prestigious job prospects in the NHS for those interested in these areas of study.

Throughout this book, I have tried my best to ensure that no false figures, facts, or statements are provided to appear to put an optimistic slant. I must therefore clarify:

1. The savings from dismantling of the NHS 111 are based on the best information I could gather. The NHS England, ONS, NHS Digital did not provide an accurate cost of running the NHS 111, requested under the Freedom of Information Act.
2. I have calculated the numbers of Psychological Wellbeing Practitioners to take over 40% of the GP appointments and Musculoskeletal Professionals to take over 30% of GP appointments, based on 20 minutes per appointment per person as compared to a standard 10-minute time for a GP appointment.

If, however, the required appointments are 30 or 40 minutes, then the number of these professionals must be increased, with good possibility of a significantly increased amount needed.

Worst case scenario:
I cannot afford the credibility of the figures I have provided above to tarnish the credibility of the book. Let us assume that the salaries of new Direct Access Psychological Welfare Professionals and Direct Access Musculoskeletal Professionals salaries, which is the foundation of my entire *revolutiq*, are doubled to provide a 40- minute appointment for each patient. In that case the salaries could be:

£ 1,892,412,000, annually x 2 = £3,784,824,000

You may remember that savings from the abolition of the NHS 111 is £1,360,000,000 and the cessation of payments based on people who do not exist is £692, 850,310, making a grand annual total of £2,052,850,310.

The maximum that the General Practice in England may need could be:

£ 3,784,824,000 minus £2,052,850,310 = £1,731,973,690
I am confident that when the revolutionary reforms are implemented, the NHS General Practice could achieve a minimum saving of 10 % from the possible budget of £15 billion. 15,000,000,000 x 10% = 1,500,000,000.

£ 1,731,973,690 minus £1,500,000,000 = £231,973,690.

A figure close to only £232 million could be required to make the NHS General Practice, one of the best in the world to provide; prompt, no-wait, face-to-face GP consultations to people during the day and same-day availability for semi-urgent problems arising after 6pm and over the weekend.

The only other alternative could be to recruit 31,065 additional GPs. (Chapter Seven)

You may remember the figures provided by NHS England, the combined salary of GP contractors and the salaried GPs is £98,000 (Chapter Five).

Cost: 31,065 GPs x £98,000 = £3,044,370,000.

This is 3 billion, 44 million, 370 thousand. Needless to say, the recruitment of 31,065 GPs is an impossibility as the NHS has discovered; unable to add even 5,000 GPs.

For the first time ever in the history of the NHS General Practice, I am offering an implementable solution, backed by facts and figures. I can say with confidence that The General

Practice Revolution would alleviate the misery of 56.5 million people in England, unable to achieve prompt GP appointments and having to face the indignity and agony of medical attention by telephone only from the despicable NHS 111.

Perhaps the greatest benefit of the General Practice Revolution would be the reversion of the prestigious A&E to a department for genuine emergencies and not for the hideous overflow of the problems created after 6pm and weekends that the GPs do not handle. This would also minimise the pressure on the Ambulance Service, created by the NHS 111 and people using their own initiative to use the service (Chapter 15).

Special note:
Number of Psychological Wellbeing Practitioners already working in the NHS General Practice in England: I have not been able to find the accurate number. According to Health Education England, Adult IAPT workforce census 2020 total number of low and high intensity staff is 8,088 and 1.17 million people entered IAPT treatment in 2019/20. (IAPT stands for Improving Access to Psychological Therapies.)

Number of Musculoskeletal Professionals already working in the NHS General Practice in England:

According to csp.org.uk, by 2018 the number of physiotherapy staff in the UK is just under 28,000.

Figures for England are not available. NHS England has already started pilot schemes in 41 areas where the Musculoskeletal Professionals (MSK) have been named 'First Contact Practitioners' to be contacted directly by patients without contacting their own GP.

Chapter Thirteen

How the General Practice Revolution would turn the tables; everyone seeking a GP's attention would transform from a 'Powerless Pawn' to a 'Valued Customer', from 'Zero to Hero'.

The outrageous absurdity of the GP receptionists trained to be practice navigators, to deter people seeking medical attention and asking the question 'why do you want to see the GP anyway?' would cease to exist. Imagine a customer wanting to buy a product or a service and being asked, 'Why do you want to buy this product from us? Please explain.'

The General Practice Revolution would communicate a new philosophy that states, 'as the customer pays our wages, the customer is king.'

A distinguished and frustrated businessman told me:

"The unsuspecting person wanting to get medical attention from a GP, is generally considered as a nuisance and treated as such by many receptionists and in some cases a patronising attitude by the GPs. They know that the people are helplessly chained to their GP practices and that their salaries and profits are guaranteed, irrespective of the exceptionally poor access to the services they provide. My company would go bust within a few weeks if this behaviour towards clients existed."

The General Practice Revolution would introduce procedures of financial incentives and disincentives to the GPs to enable those seeking Primary Care to be treated as valued customers.

You may recall one of the recommendations, where every person in England will be allocated a nominated GP (could be more than one doctor because 75 % are working part-time) (Chapter Four).

The number of persons allocated to one full-time or two part-time GPs would constitute the patients' appointments bank, from which every GP's livelihood would depend. Remember, every doctor must offer 18 appointments in one session, of which 15 must be new appointments. With reduction of the appointments by 70%, the GPs would need 'customers' wanting to make appointments with them, due to the following two proposals:

1. Any GP with fewer than 18 appointments a session will have a deduction of £10 per appointment from their salary.
2. Every GP may offer four to five extra appointments to the normal 18 and would receive £10 for every additional appointment (all these must be new patients and not repeat visits).

I have put a cap on a maximum 23 appointments in one session to avoid overburdening the doctor. Let us calculate the additional income that a GP could generate, based on just 20 additional appointments in a week.

Calculation:
20 extra appointments a week would produce an income of £200 a week (£10 x 20) 46 working weeks x 200 = £ 9,200 additional annual income.

You will agree that the possibility of making £9,200 a year by adding few more appointments in one session can be an attractive incentive. Conversely losing money because a session booked was fewer than 18 appointments is a huge disincentive.

Suddenly, the power balance changes and the person seeking a GP appointment becomes a Powerful Valued Customer.

It is important to point out that if someone's own dedicated GP is unable to offer a prompt and suitable appointment, that person would have the choice of getting an appointment with another GP. The GPs would want to attract appointments, to be able to fill a quota of 18 appointments per session and the ability to generate more income by providing appointments to additional people per session.

Let us assume that all the 26,805 GPs (to exclude registrars and locums) (NHS Digital) decide to offer just 20 additional appointments a week. Let us calculate how many brand-new appointments this financial incentive could achieve.

Calculation:
26,805 GPs x 20 additional appointments a week
= 536,100 a week.

Total new appointments over a year
46 weeks x 536,100 = 24,660,600 appointments per year.

This is 24.6 million appointments over 12 months.

I must point out that the cost of achieving these extra appointments would be:

24,660,600 x £10 = £240,606,000

Here are two calculations worthy of consideration:

Calculation number one: (surprise, surprise)

New GP appointments generated through financial incentives are 24,660.600 annually

NHS 111 offers 20,805,000 'telephone treatment consultations' annually. (Chapter Eleven)

If NHS 111 is dismantled, the surplus of GP appointments would be 24,660.600 minus 20,805,000 = 3,855,600

Calculation number Two: (greater surprise)

Please refer to Chapter Eleven where we discovered that with the new arrangements of delegating 70% of all GP appointments to the Direct Access Professionals, the new and additional GP appointments generated were 103,270,092 per year.

With the financial incentives, another 24,660,600 appointments could be created.

Grand Total: 103,270,092 plus 24,660,600 = 127,930,692 brand new face-to-face appointments annually.

NHS 111 offers 20,805,000 'telephone treatment consultations' annually as described earlier.

If the NHS 111 offering treatment by telephone only is dismantled, there would be a surplus of 127,930,692 minus 20,805,000 = 107,125,692 GP appointments annually.

The GP Practices would remain unchanged, working from the same premises, employing the same staff (manager, receptionists, nurses and, of course, the GPs) all paid for by the NHS directly instead of through the Practice. This new model of the Primary Care will constitute a team of Direct Access Professionals. (Chapter Ten)

To give credit to NHS England, several pilot schemes in England are already working in the GP practices to provide care to the people with mental health and musculoskeletal problems (Chapter Nine). Whereas the benefits of such innovation are proven, the process is too haphazard limited and random, to have any large-scale benefit to the people.

The process of diversification and centralisation of the NHS secondary care has been copied by the General Practice to merge smaller practices into large Primary Care Networks, (PCNs), erasing the concept of the family doctor but without understanding the process of specialisation and super-specialisation involved in the hospitals. If there are eight GPs in one GP practice, they do not complement each other. Each of them has the same expertise, same set of skills and offers the same service.

When once, the US President Lyndon Johnson was informed that some poor countries, backed by the then USSR were planning to join forces to compete with NATO, he retorted "zero, plus zero, plus zero, is equal to, zero". In the case of the pathetically conceived PCNs 'innovation' of involving lots of GPs in one PCN, the scenario is like Lyndon Johnson's pronouncement: 'One GP, plus one GP, plus one GP, plus one GP, (all in one PCN,) is equal to one GP.'

The General Practice revolution could add a variety of additional medical expertise, from the non-GP professionals. This would reduce the referrals to secondary care and further minimise the GP appointments for them to concentrate on the issues, which they are best suited to deal with. Just to remind you that even now 46.4 % of all GP appointments are dealt with by non-GP processionals. (BMA; Chapter Seven)

The doctors working in the General Practice seem to be an unhappy lot with a permanently low morale. Refer to Chapter Three, where we discovered the rapid drop in the number of GPs as they age. The most likely reasons are the existing GP shortages and the organisational structure where 75% of colleagues work part-time. Another factor could be the deep-seated frustration experienced by nearly 50% of the youngish 'salaried GPs', earning significantly less, working significantly more, and finding no offers of profit-sharing partnership by the GP contractors and the private companies

I had an interesting communication from a consultant physician of a teaching hospital:
"I am dismayed by the GPs whinging about the stress of their work. Unlike those of us working in hospitals, their work finishes at 6pm with no night duties, nor the weekends. I was taken aback to read a survey by King's Fund that, of 840 GP trainees, only a quarter (27%) saw themselves working full-time in General Practice. Shockingly, 51% of the respondents wanted to do 'portfolio work' after five years. This lackadaisical demeanour reflects a deep malaise and a contagion of the culture in which they are being trained. I can assure you that no such trend exists in the trainee hospital doctors, doing 30 nights a year or more, working up to 10 weekends or more over a 12-month period. The doctors being trained in General Practice, with such a negative attitude towards working in their own chosen field is highly undesirable. Could it be that they are blackmailing the NHS, because allegedly the demand for GPs hugely exceeds the supply? Or could it be that they are salivating on the rich pickings from private companies, whilst having a job and financial security from the NHS? "

I had not come across this attitude, so I decided to investigate it myself, to check the learned consultant's observations. I discovered that things were even worse. The Daily Mail reported:
"73.4 % of the male GPs wanted to work just three days a week and 74.9% of females to work three half-day sessions.

The total cost of becoming a GP is £498,489 over a ten year period."

Perhaps the time to act is when the bright youngsters full of their own importance carrying a mountain of A stars are offered a university placement. They should be informed as a condition of the admission to a medical school, they must enter into a legally binding contract. The contract should stipulate that they would work full-time for a period of seven years minimum after entering the profession as a GP or after appointment as a consultant. At the expiry of this period, they can continue to work for the NHS or resign and work for the private companies; not both. Anyone not happy with the arrangement, can chose a different profession.

Remember what Paul Krugman the Nobel prize economist said "Productivity is not everything but in the long term it is almost everything. A country's ability to improve its standard of living depends almost entirely on its ability to raise its output per worker"

The NHS General Practice Revolution would significantly improve productivity of the GPs through the well proven system of financial incentives and at the same time making the end users as valued customers.

Chapter Fourteen

NHS England boasts: "The General Practice is undeniably the bedrock of NHS care; GPs have one of the highest public satisfaction ratings of any public service."

Healthwatch England says: "About 75% people were reporting negative experience with accessing GP services".

As I was progressing in my research into General Practice, I was constantly surprised by the rosy picture that NHS England had continued to present through the Ipsos Mori GP Patient Survey. The findings of three consecutive years have been widely quoted indicating the General Practice as a success story.

"The majority of individuals, 81.8%, rated their overall experience of their GP practice as good. Around 65.5% rated their overall experience making an appointment as good. 65.2% said it was easy to get through their GP Practice on the phone." (NHS England))

My research findings are totally contrary to these findings, including Boris Johnson's famous pronouncement, "My job is to make sure you don't have to wait for three weeks to see your GP."

How can a Primary Care Service which takes two weeks or more to even access it, offers 110 hours a week of all GP treatment by phone only, through a call centre, possibly have 81.8 % positive rating by the people of England?

I decided to request a survey, from the two reputable companies, ICM Unlimited and Survation (kind courtesy of the Charity 'Save Nation's Health')

ICM Unlimited Survey Question

The average waiting time for a GP appointment is two weeks (according to a survey of GPs conducted by Pulse Today). Which of the following statements best reflects your view on this?

The results were:

Two weeks is an acceptable amount of time to wait - 19 %
Two weeks is not an acceptable amount of time to wait - 75 %
Don't know - 6%

SURVATION Survey Question

In the UK, the average waiting time for a GP appointment is around two weeks. Which of the following statements best reflects your view on this?

The results were:

Two weeks is an acceptable amount of time to wait for a GP appointment   - 16 %

2 weeks is not an acceptable amount of time to wait for a GP appointment   - 79%

Don't know   - 5%

It was interesting to note that when asked a direct question if the waiting time to see a GP for two weeks was acceptable, the overwhelming majority said that it was not. The two responses of 75 % and 79%, as unacceptable in the survey conducted by two reputable companies related to waiting are very relevant.

I decided to do some research on the baffling contradictions of the NHS England survey by Ipsos Mori and the two independent companies commissioned by the charity 'Save

Nation's Health'. I requested a university lecturer with a special interest in the social surveys to please investigate the matter and give his independent view. This is what she said:

"The pay-masters of an organisation, wanting a certain outcome from a public survey can achieve their objective by slanting questions to evoke a favourable response. We all know that waiting time to get a GP appointment of two weeks or more has been widely published and criticised by the media, the people and even the UK Prime Minister. However, a question relating to it has never been asked by Mori, in collaboration with NHS England.

The finding of 81.8%, of people rating their overall experience of their GP practice as good and 65.5% rating their overall experience making an appointment as good, appears to have deliberately avoided the question, as asked by ICM Unlimited and Survation. This question elicited an overwhelming response of 75% and 79% from people stating that two weeks waiting to secure a GP appointment is not acceptable.

Imagine an Amazon Survey of a coffee machine where 90 % of people give 5 stars to the experience of fast delivery, beautiful packaging, attractive colour, ease of use. However, 98% people give it one star, stating that the coffee the machine makes is dreadful and the experience of drinking is awful.

In my opinion, the Mori GP Patient Survey is Amazon's coffee machine survey. The question which would have likely to produce a 90 % response of awful, was never asked. I was surprised to note that in its PR campaign to announce the approval rating of General Practice, it does not state that out of all the people who were surveyed, 69.3 % of people who were sent questionnaires did not participate in the survey. The favourable results were obtained from a minority of 31.7%

respondents, asking their experience and not their verdict of a two-week wait for an appointment."

The fact remains that 69.3% respondents decided not to participate in the survey.

On a separate note, NHS England's tendency to make announcements which turn out to be false, erode its credibility.

"By March 2018, the mandate requires that 40% of the country will benefit from extended access to GP appointments at evenings and weekends, but we are aiming for 50% by March 2019 this will extend to 100% of the country.'   (NHS Five Year Forward View Key Improvements 2017/18 and 2018/19; NHS England)

After more than three years this has not materialised.

Chapter Fifteen

The two weeks wait to get a GP appointment and dissatisfaction of treatment by telephone from NHS 111, drives people to the Accident and Emergency departments turning them to General Practice Surgeries. This destabilises the entire secondary care system - living proof of the undeniable incompetence of the NHS management.

In the previous chapters I have explained how helpless people, unable to get a GP appointment, dismayed by the telephone treatment from the notorious NHS 111, flock to A&E departments to wait for hours for a face-to-face consultation.

"People will go to A&E if there is nowhere else to go, and their condition may deteriorate leading to increased treatment and care because they couldn't get help sooner.
(Sir Robert Francis, Chairman, Healthwatch England)

It's become such a common course of action to use A&E in this way, that it's even filtered through to TV programmes. A friend sent me photos from a television series which appear to indicate that the GP practices now consider A&E as a logical part and parcel of Primary Care. By incorporating this message into TV programmes, it sends a signal to viewers that this is what they should do if they're unable to get a GP appointment.

Here is the transcript of the recording from the live popular TV series of a GP practice (GPs Behind Closed Doors)

Telephonist to the patient: "you're saying that your body hurts or aches? Normally, the practice is to go to A&E"

Practice nurse after checking the blood pressure, to the patient: "I am just going to run it past the doctor".

Practice nurse to the GP: "It's the patient I've been seeing for his blood pressure, he's 39. I've done his blood pressure today."

GP: "What were the readings like?"

Practice nurse: "175 over 125"

Practice nurse returns to the patient and speaks to him: "So, I have spoken to the doctor because of the headaches and how high your blood pressure is. You need to head down to A&E".

Patient: "A&E?"

Practice Nurse: "What they'll probably do is just monitor it for a bit. And if comes down, then fine, but if not, they probably will want to investigate why it's so…so high".

GP to the patient: "The best course of action would be for you to go to A&E".

Patient to his wife: "And (the GP) said that if it hadn't gone down substantially within 48 hours, to go to A&E. Yeah."

The cumulative effect of people's inability to get prompt GP appointments, dissatisfaction with the telephone NHS 111 treatment and GPs' encouragement to seek medical advice from the A&E departments, leads to an unacceptable work overload.

"A&E doctors across the country revealed that in some units, people are waiting as long as nine hours to be seen.' (The Daily Independent newspaper)

"The levels of increase in A&E's activity is creating a significant and sustained threat to patient safety. Research evidence has consistently demonstrated that excessive

occupancy in emergency departments is inevitably associated with an increase in short term mortality. The essence of emergency medicine is identifying the needle in the haystack. If the haystack gets bigger, it becomes progressively bigger to find the needle."
(Dr. Adrian Boyle, Vice President, Royal College of Emergency Medicine)

My interviews with several A&E consultants indicate that 30-40% of all attendances are neither an accident nor an emergency and could have been dealt with by the GPs.

What surprises me most is the inability of the NHS Management to find the root cause of this catastrophe when a learned doctor has been forced to compare the people attending the Emergency Departments as a haystack and finding a genuine emergency a needle. I must hasten to add that the increasingly growing number of people in the A&E departments is not an alleged abuse. No one could have put it more eloquently and accurately than Sir Robert Francis: 'People will go to A&E if there is nowhere else to go.'

What I have advocated in this book is a solution to the daily sufferings of the people forced to build haystacks and the stresses of the doctors desperately trying to find the 'needles'. Minimising the GP appointments to 30%, abolishing the NHS 111 and making availability of face-to-face consultations from the GPs after 6 pm and the weekends, would put an end to this situation.

We, the English people are not dim, not abusers of systems. Give us the dignity to have medical attention from the GPs when we need it, after 6 pm, on weekends, promptly and with compassion, not forcing us to lie on trollies in the corridors of A&E for hours as if it was a war zone in an African country.

Let the hard-working doctors in A&E deal with genuine accidents and emergencies.

Chapter Sixteen

Story of the Unclaimed £10,000 REWARD

As the research of the book was in progress I decided to "put my money, where my mouth is' and sent an individually addressed letter to influential members of the four health-related Think Tanks. The list of the names of the people the letter was sent to is at the end of this chapter.

This is a copy of the letter I wrote:

I invite you to win: **£10,000 REWARD**, if you can prove that: The General Practice in England is ACCEPTABLE as an Essential Public Sector Service, considering:

- GPs provide treatment to their registered patients for 30% of the time only in any one week. (Monday to Friday, 8am to 6pm.)
- The remaining 70% of the problems of the registered patients, are left to be treated by telephone, through the Call Centre NHS 111
- People are forced to wait two weeks for a GP appointment.
- The General Practice operates 'for profit' by the self-employed GP contractors and the private companies.

You have my personal guarantee, that the reward sum is available and would be paid, in accordance with the fair and equitable terms and conditions,

Yours sincerely

Dr. Hamid Sarwar

Some Facts & Figures

The average national waiting time to get a GP appointment is two weeks. (Survey, GPs magazine PULSE)

'My job is to make sure; you don't have to wait three weeks to see your GP,' (Speech by Boris Johnson, 24 July 2019.)

'One GP earned, £600,000 - £700,000 in pensionable pay.
Another received   £500,000 - £600,000.
A further 14 were paid   £300,000 - £400,000,
with 146 earning   £200,000 - £300,000.
Nearly 5,500 earned   £100,000 - £200,000.
(PA Press Association, Nick McDermott, The Sun, 5 January 2020.)

GPs offer appointments 8am -6pm, Monday to Friday only. The rest of the Primary Care is provided through '24/7 telephone call centres 111' by medically unqualified people with six weeks' training. Please see Trust Pilot reviews on the quality of service provided by the 111.

At the time of writing more than 35 private companies are registered to provide General Practice in England, many promising a next-day appointment (on payment) with NHS GPs, who are unable to see their own patients for two weeks.

The impressive list of some international inventors in the General Practice; Swedish Investment Group AB Kinnevik, BXR group, Demis Hassabis and Mustafa Suleyman, Hoxton ventures, Sawiris, NNS Holdings, Vostok New Ventures, Saudi Arabia's Public Investment Fund, Munich Re's ERGO Fund, the US based Centene corporation, Livi, Boots.

Simple Terms & Conditions to claim the £10,000 REWARD

1. Please post your Reward Claim Document by post, to the address or email provided.
2. There is no limit to the number of words or pages.
3. The Reward Claim Document will be examined by a panel of three independent individuals for approval, on an objective basis.
4. In the case of rejection of the claim, a detailed letter or email would be sent to the claimant on why the Reward Claim may have been rejected. An appeal may be lodged, which would be reviewed by a panel of three independent people headed by a barrister. The decision of the panel would be final but can be challenged through an independent panel of arbitration.
5. The reward money would be equally distributed if there are more than one successful claimant, by the deadline date for submission.
6. The Reward Claim must be submitted by no later than (date) and sent to:

Email address and postal address both provided

A list of people to whom the £10,000 REWARD Invitation letter was sent:

The Health Foundation:
Sir Hugh Taylor. David Smart. Sharmila Nebhrajani. Dr Ruth Hussey CB OBE, Eric Gregory. Loraine Hawkins. Professor Rosalind Smyth CBE. Branwen Jeffreys, Melloney Poole OBE, Martyn Hole. Sir David Dalton. Dr Jennifer Dixon, Aidan Kearney, Will Warburton, Adam Steventon, Anita Charlesworth, Cathy Irving, Jo Bibby.

Nuffield Health:

Steve Gray. Chris Blackwell-Frost, Caroline Smith, Jenny Dillon, Martin Friend, Jane Garvey, Dr Natalie-Jane Macdonald, Lord Victor Adebowale, Martin Bryant, Patrick Figgis, Dame Lin Homer, David Lister, Steve Mason, Neil Sachdev MBE.

The King's Fund:

Rt. Hon. Professor Ajay Kakkar, Alex Bayliss, Alison Trimble, Amanda Wilsher, Andrew McCracken, Andrew Willis, Angela Coulter, Anna Charles, Dr Aseem Malhotra, Becca Shepard, Beccy Baird, Belinda Weir, Ben Collins. Ben Fuchs, Caroline Viac, Dr Carolyn Wilkins OBE, Chloe Smithers, Chris Naylor, Clair Thorstensen-Woll, Claire Perry, Claire Taylor, Clare Sutherland, Dan Wellings, Danielle Roche, Dave Thornton, David Buck, David Fillingham CBE, David Maguire, David Naylor, David Oliver, Deborah Fenney, Deborah Homer.

20/20 Health:

Julia Manning, Kathy Mason, Matt James, Jon Paxman, Dame Helena Shovelton, Andrew Burns, Dr Paul Hodgkin, Richard Lucas, Dr Mark Martin, Barbara Arzymanow, Gail Beer, Angel Thompson MBE, Professor Nigel Cameron, Iseult Roche, Drew Provan, Lisa Rodrigues CBE, Mo Girach, Kevin J Dean, David Pascall CBE, John Bowis OBE.

Not Surprisingly, to date, no one has claimed the reward.

Chapter Seventeen

Your GP Will See You Now (by telephone, in two weeks)

Face-to face consultation, followed by physical examination are the two unchanged fundamentals of doctors' protocol to undertake further investigations, if necessary, make a diagnosis and commence treatment. The GPs in England were quick to stop seeing their patients, as soon the pandemic started and offered diagnosis and treatment through telephone only.

Eighty percent of GPs say that a return to pre-pandemic levels of face-to-face appointments is not necessary". (Survey by the GPs publication Pulse)

Fury, as the Chair of the Royal College of GPs says. "Patients will get used to not seeing their GP face to face. (Headline, the Daily Mail)

Virtual consultations are unsafe:
"As a doctor seeing patients in person can give you vital clinical clues. It is sad so many appointments have gone online because you can miss important health information, and this can be unsafe." (Queens former doctor Sir Richard Thompson)

An acquaintance told me:
" I have been unable to get a non- telephone appointment from any of the four GPs partners in the practice since March 2020 right up to December 2021. I am full of gratitude, to the wonderful doctors who have helped me in the A&E. Waiting for more than four hours on each occasion to be seen, I did not mind. It probably saved my life. Throughout this period, the people in my local supermarket have served me along with hundreds of others. What is the problem with the GPs? They

are a disgrace to the profession. Is there no-one to check them?"

A mother-of-three said:
" Pubs and restaurants now have dozens of people sitting and eating, TV shows hundreds of people dancing in the night clubs. The double-vaccinated GPs and their double-vaccinated staff were too scared to give my seven-year-old daughter a face-to-face appointment for fear of alleged safety of their patients. Please, forgive me for saying it, but their professional behaviour has been disgusting since the pandemic and explains why many surgeries have had graffiti painted over and why many GPs and their staff are facing daily abuse."

Strong words but these statements appear to represent the public outrage, as shown by the various national newspapers:

Coroner raises the alarm over remote GPs after six deaths:
"Remote GP appointments may have been a contributing factor in the deaths of five people who did not see their doctor face-to-face a coroner has concluded. Alison Mutch, senior coroner for Greater Manchester South has asked Health Secretary Sajid Javid and NHS England to tackle risks associated with remote appointments, a Health Service Journal investigation found". (The Daily Telegraph)

Virtual GP visits are 'costing lives :
"Tensions are growing between GPs and hospital doctors, who say signs of illness, such as breast cancer are being missed due to the lack of a physical examination. It comes as accident and emergency departments are under increasing pressure, with patients frequently being referred to hospital without first having an in-person examination by their GPs." (Rosamund Urwin, Tom Calver, Caroline Wheeler, The Sunday Times)

Nazi B***ds:**

GPs facing torrent of abuse and violence as patient frustrations boil over. Doctors and their staff working across England are reporting a torrent of abuse from patients with some receiving hate mail. Some surgeries have been subjected to bomb threats while others have been daubed with graffiti. A London GP practice received this pamphlet:

WARNING
TO ALL MEDICAL PRACTITIONERS
DOCTORS AND NURSES
"I was just carrying out orders"
Is **NOT** a legal defence
YOU WILL BE ON TRIAL FOR WAR CRIMES
& HELD ACCOUNTABLE
(The Independent, newspaper)

A betrayal of the NHS. The only people GPs are keeping healthy with their scandalous refusal to meet patients face-to-face are themselves.

"The real scandal is happening at GP surgeries all over the country. Waiting rooms lie empty, lines of freshly sanitised chairs sit without occupants. Signs on external doors say 'do not enter without appointment'- so the sick stay at home and potentially shorten their lives, forced to hang on to the phone waiting for ages or try log on, remember their NHS number, password and navigate a complicated website. It is easier for Michel Gove to enter a night club mask-less, than it is to meet your local GP face-to face. As a result of the reduction in face-face consultations, the lack of cancer diagnosis means the UK's cancer survival rates have dropped to between ten to fifteen years BEHIND comparable countries
(Janet Street Porter, The Daily Mail)

When will the GPs go back to working normally again?
"By normal I mean, seeing their patients in flesh, looking in ears and down throats, palpating stomachs, examining lumps, manipulating lumps, these and all the procedures part of a face-to-face appointment? Dentists have been back in their surgeries, staring in their patients mouths for months. Physiotherapists and osteopaths are seeing people flat out. You can have your eyebrows waxed, your toes manicured, have your hair done. M&S will even fit a bra for you, but GPs still won't routinely encounter their patients in the flesh." (Joanna Blythman, columnist)

Nearly 1,000 GP surgeries in England are ordered to provide more face-to-face appointments, to 'get a grip' on growing number of patients struggling to see a doctor in person. NHS England identified more than 900 practices that are failing to meet basic standard patient access, with long waiting times and low levels of satisfaction. (dailymail.co.uk)

75% of them face abuse every day, including assaults, threats, racism, and sexism. A recent poll by the body representing GP surgery staff across the UK.
(The Institute of General Practice Management)

Generous GP pay isn't working for patients!
"The poorest and sickest are neglected as many doctors opt to practice part-time in affluent areas and then retire early. The love of money is the root of all evil, but it can be quite useful too. Used in the right way and the right place, the lure of wealth can motivate people to do good and necessary. Get it wrong, though, and the power of money creates big problems. Just ask a doctor, if you can see one".
(James Kirkup, The Times)

If the GPs went on strike, would anyone notice? :
"The British Medical Association annual meeting will take place next week. In view of the almost universal dissatisfaction of General Practice and in order to prove to the public that yet more taxpayer money would be wasted on service that deliver little to the patients, I would suggest that an emergency motion be tabled: 'This meeting recommends the radical reform of primary care'… the case for reform is particularly strong for primary care. The system has been irreversibly damaged because some GPs have been allowed to run it for their own convenience and not for the benefit of their patients". (J. Merion Thomas, The Telegraph)

Campaign to make GPs see all patients face-to-face again.
"The new regime has led to vast swathes of patients feeling all but abandoned by their family doctors, according to more than 1,000 letters and emails received by this newspaper over the past eight months. We are calling for health chiefs to change their guidance and reopen GP Surgeries before it threatens to cause a spiralling crisis". (Mail on Sunday)

Almost 1,000 GP practices have been ordered to improve patient access, amid growing concerns about the number of patients struggling to see a family doctor. (The Telegraph)

I asked an eminent consultant physician working in a renowned teaching hospital to give his opinion on GPs' insistence to offer consultations by phone and that people must get used to not seeing their GP face-to-face, as announced by the chair of the Royal College of GPs.

He said:

"I have practiced medicine for 15 years as a consultant. I am shocked and appalled and unable to understand the reasoning behind the GPs wanting to continue to offer treatment by telephone. I believe it is nearly impossible to make a diagnosis without physical examination. This is so fundamental to medicine that no doctor anywhere in the world can support treatment through telephone (except, it appears, GPs in England). What is the advantage to GPs in treating people by telephone? They are unlikely to offer treatment to a greater number of patients. They and their staff have received double jabs. I have been seeing and treating patients throughout the pandemic; at a time, no vaccines were available. Soldiers must face the enemy to risk their life; the doctors must face pandemics and risk their life. It appears that GPs in England would rather risk the lives of their patients."

The NHS General Practice Revolution Promise:
The fundamental criterion of doctor's face-to-face consultations, followed by clinical examinations to decide on further investigations, diagnosis and treatment would be restored. Treatment through telephone would be abolished.

Grand Summary of The General Practice Revolution.

The General Practice in England is a fundamentally flawed operational model. No amount of cash or misguided reforms can change it from what is now universally acknowledged as one of the worst in the world for GP access. The book has identified the problems that have led to the system's near-collapse and provides a straightforward solution to how this can be reversed operationally and financially through the General Practice Revolution.

Problems:

1. The average waiting time to get a GP appointment is two weeks. Out of 168 hours a week, the GPs are available only for 50 hours (Monday to Friday 8 am-6 pm). England is the only rich country in the world where for 118 hours a week, people are offered treatment by telephone from a call centre, the NHS 111. Operated by 'Health Advisers' with no medical qualification and six weeks of training, the NHS 111 is considered a disaster by people who have used it (Chapter Five).

2. Those unable to get GP appointments or dissatisfied by receiving treatment by phone from the NHS 111 rush to the A&E departments, which have now become GP surgeries. The vast number of people who could have been efficiently dealt with by the GPs overwhelm the A & E departments causing severe delays in dealing with genuine emergencies destabilising the Secondary Care.

3. Though funded entirely by the taxpayers, the General Practice in England is a commercial enterprise owned by the self-employed GPs called GP contractors, who run it for profit. They constitute less than 50% of the total GPs' workforce but employ the rest as salaried

doctors, locums, trainee registrars and more than 100,000 practice staff. Some can earn up to five times more than the PM.

4. The NHS is short of 31,065 full-time GPs or a staggering 98,241 if the current practice of part-timers is continued. (Chapter Seven).

5. GP practices have 4.47 million patients on their list, who do not exist and are called ghost patients and for which they receive £692.85 million annually.

6. Seventy-five per cent of the GPs work part-time.

7. GPs continue to insist on providing treatment by telephone, though triple vaccinated and long after the pandemic, causing huge outcry and resentment from the public and the press.

Solutions:

1. The sham self-employed status of the GPs would be abolished, making them salaried doctors and an employee like all the other doctors working for the NHS. Hundreds of millions of pounds of profits made by the GP contractors and the private companies will be saved and invested back to the General Practice. Ghost patients would cease to exist, adding back in excess of £690 million every year.

2. Forty per cent of all the GP appointments are about mental health issues and 30% are for musculoskeletal conditions. The General Practice Revolution would offer 40 % of all the mental health problems to Psychological Wellbeing Practitioners and 30% to Musculoskeletal Practitioners, through Direct Access and without a GP consultation. Several well-documented studies based on trials show outstanding and better outcomes for people with mental health problems and those with pain in muscles, bones and

joints when treated by the Direct Access Professionals than with the involvement of the GPs.

3. For the first time in the seventy years of history of the NHS, the role of the GPs as the first point of contact would be reduced to 30%, dealing with medical matters only. The remaining 70% would be dealt with by Direct Access Professionals, without a GP appointment. (Details in Chapter Nine and Key Points of the book.) There is proven evidence of superior clinical outcomes with this arrangement.

Abolition of the self-employed status of the GP contractors, dismantling the NHS 111, diverting 70 % of all GP appointments by direct access to non-GP professionals would provide 24/7 face-to-face, prompt, hassle-free treatment to everyone. **This is the NHS General Practice Revolution.**

Implementing detailed strategies and plans in the book, The General Practice in England would become 'pride of the nation and the envy of the world'. It will be 'the duty of the NHS to protect the people, and not that of the people to protect the NHS.

Key Points of the NHS General Practice Revolution

GPs' working hours are like that of a bank manager.
Apart from England, there is no other rich country in which the entire population is denied face-to-face consultations with a GP, after 6 pm and at weekends, and delegated to a telephone call centre. (110 hours a week out of 168.) GPs are ostensibly available 8 am to 6 pm, but the average waiting for an appointment is two weeks.

The call centre NHS 111, offering treatment for 110 hours a week out of 168 by telephone, staffed by Health Advisers with no medical qualification would be dismantled.
The Covid-19 Bereaved Families for Justice Group believes that several hundred of its members had a relative die after calling 111 and being told that they should stay at home. A probe by The Healthcare Safety Investigation Branch (HSIB) is in progress.

The GP contractors.
The General Practice in England, though entirely funded by the taxpayers, is owned by the self-employed GPs called GP contractors, who run it for profit. They constitute less than 50% of the total GPs workforce but employ the rest as salaried doctors, locums, trainee registrars, and more than 100,000 of England's practice staff. Apart from seniority and good luck, they do not possess any extra qualifications and can earn a profit of between £110,000 to £700,000 annually. In addition, a small and increasing number of private companies have joined the money-making bandwagon.

The sham self-employed status of the GP contractors would be abolished, all GPs paid salaries, like their hospital colleagues.
NHS England will take back control and appoint more GPs in

poorer areas of England. For example, GPs are 54 per 100,000 people in Northwest London compared to 69 per 100,000 in South West. The GPs would be obliged to work some weekends and after 6 pm like their hospital colleagues. Every person in England would be allocated a nominated and dedicated GP. The traditional family doctor system would be restored.

Only 25% of GPs work full-time.

An astonishing 75% of the permanent GPs work part-time only, just 25% work full-time. Nevertheless, part-time workers in England constitute 25% of the total workforce.

GP Shortages. No-one knows how many, and no-one has ever found out.

NHS England, fully supported by the academics of the Royal College of General Practitioners, advocates of the British Medical Association, stars of the NHS related think tanks, and the politicians, all agree that a shortage of GPs is one of the major problems facing the General Practice in England. Shortage figures of 5,000 - 9,000 are brandished. No-one knows how many. And no-one has ever found out. In this book, I have done so.

The BOMBSHELL.

The General Practice in England is short of 31,065 full-time GPs and a staggering number of 98,241 additional GPs if the decade's old current practice of 75% doctors working part-time in the NHS General Practice is maintained. NHS England has been unable to add even 5,000 GPs in 5 years!

Further progress of the book stopped for five months.

I could not find a solution to overcome the GP shortage catastrophe exposed by my research.

The Eureka Breakthrough.

Disappointed and in a state of utter despair, one day, out of the blue, I made a discovery which made me cry, 'Eureka!'.

- 40% of all the GP appointments are about mental health problems
- 30% of GP appointments are for musculoskeletal conditions.

The General Practice in England should offer 40 % of all the mental health problems to Psychological Wellbeing Practitioners and 30% to Musculoskeletal Practitioners, through Direct Access, and without a GP consultation. Several well-documented studies based on trials show outstanding and better outcomes for people with mental health problems and those with pain in muscles, bones and joints when treated by the Direct Access Professionals without the involvement of the GPs.

For the first time ever, the role of the GP as the first contact will be reduced to 30%.

This would solve once for all shortage of GPs and when helped by the existing Advance Nurse Practitioners the NHS requires only 12,282 full-time GPs. (Chapter Nine)

GP practices have 4.47 million patients on their list who do not exist and are called ghost patients, for which they receive £ 692.85 million annually.

Chapter 12 explains how a modest sum of £232 million could be needed to recruit all the Direct Access Professionals by the money saved from the exorcism of ghost patients, dismantling of the NHS 111 and other actions.

Finding needles in a haystack.

"The essence of emergency medicine is identifying the needle

in the haystack. If the haystack gets bigger, it becomes progressively bigger to find the needle."
(Dr. Adrian Boyle, Vice President, RCEM)

When people can access GPs without waiting during the day, after 6 pm and at the weekends, it would end creating the daily haystacks from where the doctors are trying to find needles. The A&E's will cease to be treated as GP surgeries and restored to genuine emergency departments. Interviews with several A&E consultants indicate that 30-40% of all attendances are neither an accident nor an emergency and could have been dealt with by the GPs.

Other Important Matters.
All that a GP needs to perform his duties is a consulting room with a hand wash sink, an examination couch, a doctor's chair, a desk for a computer, two chairs for the patients, all housed in an eight square meter room. Believe it or not, that's it.

Currently, 46.4% of all GP appointments are dealt with by non-GP healthcare professionals.

There is no evidence that GPs deliver a superior quality of consultations from the opulent health centres costing millions compared to those working from humble, old surgery premises.

The GPs, full-time or part-time, will be given a choice to work for the NHS or the private companies, **not** both.

With a reduction of all GP appointments to 30%, the incentive and disincentive scheme will turn people seeking GP treatment from powerless pawns to valued customers.

The distressing experience of waiting for hours on the phone to get an appointment will be replaced by the online appointment system, with contact facilities on the phone for those with no internet access.

A survey from two reputable companies found that "75% and 79% of people believe that two weeks is not an acceptable amount of time to wait for a GP appointment." (Findings from ICM and Survation, respectively.)

All the GPs, serving the private companies and offering instant appointments but unable to offer an NHS appointment for two weeks to their reregistered patients are fully-paid NHS GPs, with six weeks' holidays, gold-plated pension schemes and sick pay benefits. Such NHS GPs say "No, we cannot offer you an appointment for 2 weeks from our NHS practice, but if you are prepared to pay us through a private company, yes, we are at your service, now"!

Politicians, academics and some left-wing activists have been worrying and protesting about the threat of 'the NHS General Practice Privatisation'. The fact is that the NHS General Practice in England is a commercial enterprise, run for profit by the GP contractors and the private companies. National and international investors see the General Practice in England as a golden opportunity to make money.

At the heart of the *revolutiq* is a 'turnaround' of the existing system:

- Abolish the self-employed status of the GPs. Everyone to have a dedicated GP.
- Introduce direct access non-GP professionals to let the GPs deal with the medical problems only, constituting 30 % of all appointments.
- Allow people to consult direct access Psychological Wellbeing Practitioners and direct access Musculoskeletal Practitioners (70% of consultations) without the GPs.
- Dismantle the NHS 111 providing 110 hours/week treatment by telephone.
- Treat everyone using the General Practice as a valued customer.
- Reinvest into the General Practice the profits made by the GP contractors, the private companies, and the ghost patients.

Funded 100% by the taxpayers, the NHS General Practice would cease to be a money-making machine and would be run for the benefit of the people it is meant to serve and not for the benefit of its employees.

The NHS General Practice Revolution would create prompt, no-wait, face-to-face, 24/7 GP consultations for the people during the day, same-day availability for semi-urgent and urgent problems arising after 6 pm and over the weekends. The admirable and traditional concept of the family doctor will be restored.

EPILOGUE

Treatment Delayed is Treatment Denied

The two reasons to write a book are 'to get famous or make a lot of money. My motivation is neither. All the royalties are to go to the charity 'Save Nation's Health'. I have no desire or illusion of becoming famous.

My reason for writing the book is to change the appalling system of General Practice we have in England. Unfortunately, the book may sell well without having the slightest impact on how the General Practice in England continues to damage the physical and mental health of the people and inflict misery, pain and suffering.

If a charity asked for donations to help the population of a developing country because no medical attention was available without waiting for fourteen days and 70% of the time the treatment was available by telephone only, the people in England would give generously to the cause. And yet, unknown to most, this is how the General Practice is available to us in our own country.

People who have not needed medical assistance in England continue to believe in the myth that "the NHS is the pride of the nation and envy of the world". Those who have the misfortune to use the General Practice are in a state of helplessness and misery, not knowing what to do except suffering in silence. Brainwashed over decades, they are doomed to accept that "it is the duty of everyone to protect the NHS".

The clever managers of the NHS have successfully convinced every Government that the General Practice is the bedrock of the NHS, enjoys massive popularity by the public and has no significant problem except GP shortages. The ministers meekly shut up at the mention of more funds.

The operational and financial model of the NHS General Practice is so fundamentally flawed that only a 'revolution' can change it. This 'revolution' will not happen by the simple act of publication of the book. The 'revolution' will only happen if the Prime Minister and the MPs read the book, accept its findings, decide to act and implement the recommendations through legislation.

The book offers a detailed, evidence-based plan of action to provide people of England a 'no wait', hassle-free, face-to-face GP consultations 24/7/365. How can anyone possibly argue with it? Especially when no extra funding is required except a modest and affordable sum.

It becomes evident that the only way to bring about a 'revolution' in the NHS General Practice is to convince the Government in power that people in England should receive the same level of primary care as is available in almost every rich country. My research indicates that it can only be achieved through a 'campaign' to persuade the decision-makers in the Government in power. The book can act as a 'campaign manual' to demonstrate the clarity of the implementable proposals.

I am aware of several campaigns that have helped change the world's social and political landscape in the last 150 years. However, my study on the subject reveals that with some notable exceptions, most campaigns fail to achieve their goal and, in some cases, can attract public resentment and hostility.

I am no campaigner. I need help, your help. So, I will start the ball rolling by taking the first step by writing about the book to the Prime Minister, The Health Secretary and all the MPs of England, requesting them to please pay attention and act. This would be a long and continuous process aimed directly at all the MPs through various communication channels.

The next step would be to reach out to both print and digital media to include newspapers, social media and the various TV channels to try to influence those who could influence the influencers.

The most crucial support would be from you. As stated earlier, many people in England are still unaware of how disastrous the General Practice is. So, I need your help as volunteers to join forces together in a structured way to help change what must be changed, for you, your family, your friends, and all of us.

Please get in touch with me and tell me how you can help? Please do. Thank you.

contact@nhsrevolution.org

A website has been set up to help the campaign and will have regular updates to include your inputs. www.nhsrevolution.org

The NHS General Practice Revolution Concludes:

- It is the duty of the NHS General Practice to protect the people, not the duty of the people to protect the NHS General Practice.

- The NHS General Practice should be meant for the benefit of the people using it and not for the benefit of those working in it, as appears to be the case now.

- Implementing the recommendations of the book, 'no-wait', face-to-face, 24/7 GP consultations are achievable.

Reviews

The NHS General Practice Revolution is a hard-hitting, and very timely, polemic that addresses the crisis within the GP system and makes carefully weighed and costed suggestions for how to fix it within existing budget constraints. The author has drawn on his experience as a GP to comment on the present arrangements, concluding that they are wholly inadequate, the cause of widespread public dissatisfaction, and often lead to harmful, even fatal outcomes when people cannot obtain prompt appointments. The NHS is a perennial hot-button political issue, unfailingly taking centre-stage at most general elections. The book is an impressive achievement in showing that problems seen by government as too costly, by users as too administratively intractable to solve, are entirely addressable if the political will for a radical overhaul could be mustered.

So often these debates are couched in terms of the eternal stand-off between campaigners and opposition politicians demanding that more be done, and governments defensively insisting that the economy cannot afford it, but the author has valiantly cut through this impasse by framing the argument in explicitly economic terms. The many statistical calculations that punctuate the text confer a professional authority on it that goes beyond the mere articulating of wish-lists, which always plays into the hands of the Treasury. Suffice to say that I learned something new from every chapter of the book and was repeatedly fascinated by the various findings – such as the analysis of what problems people present to GPs with, how little essential equipment and working space the surgeries genuinely need, and the manifold commercial embroilments that obtain between contractors and the private sector.

Stuart Walton is a cultural historian, critical theorist and novelist. Author of several books including: *An Excursion Through Chaos; In the Realm of the Senses; A Natural History of Human Emotions; The First Day in Paradise; Out of It: A Cultural History of Intoxication; and many more.*

Inside back page

a

The book explains the urgent need for GP reform in no uncertain terms, all backed with documented research. Most importantly it offers a simple solution. Why is it not happening? Having experienced 1st hand, the difficulties described by the book in using GP and NHS111 Services whilst looking after my 91-year-old mother-in-law, I have to agree the primary care service has become totally dysfunctional.

The book is an interesting read and points out the brainwashing that goes on to convince us that it is "our NHS" - it is not! It is for the benefit of those exploiting the system and milking loopholes that should have been closed decades ago. And as for the envy of the world, try Spain, Thailand, Japan, France and many other countries that beat us in the world rankings. At the last time of looking, we had fallen to 15th.

The book quite rightly points out, why is it the GP contractor is exempt from IR35 when lorry drivers and a lot of other subcontractors have had this status forcibly removed by HMRC!

Businesses realised decades ago that to survive and prosper they must put their customer 1st. Unfortunately, the NHS GP's customer, the patient, to date has not! Most shockingly of all, no company in the world allows its employees to work part time so that they can moonlight for a competitor, unbelievable!

This book is a must read to allow you to understand the problems in detail and how simple it would be to correct with huge savings. The government must act now!

Steve Bristow was the CEO and now the chairman of a successful company operating for over thirty years. His innovation and forward thinking have won plaudits from his peers

This book is an eye opener about the true state of General practice in the UK.

I was surprised to note that the General Practice in England, though entirely funded by the NHS, is owned by less than 50% of the GPs workforce called GP contractors, who run it for profit and employ other GPs as salaried doctors at significantly less salary than their own profits. More surprising to find that these GP contractors are self-employed. I cannot employ persons as self-employed if they work exclusively and for any length of time for the company. The HMRC legislation of IR35 has been introduced to stop people avoiding tax and NI when in effect they are employed and not self-employed. How do the GP contractors get away with it? The book highlights the serious issues and gives real solutions to address them.

Mr. Paul Farmer OBE is the Managing Director of Wade Ceramics. The company employs more than 200 people. He has been awarded an honorary doctorate for playing a 'significant role' in regeneration of the city

Inside back page

c

Printed in Great Britain
by Amazon

20031267R00081